I believe there is much to learn about APD, much to understand. I also believe there is much to celebrate on behalf of our children.

—Karen J. Foli

LIKE SOUND THROUGH WATER

"Read this book as you would a novel, a story about discovery and disappointment, understanding and misunderstanding, learning and not learning, hope and despair, and love in the face of difficult times, love that never, never quits."

—Edward M. Hallowell, M.D.

"Karen's story has meant the world to me."

—A parent in Wisconsin

"This book has somehow made my family's journey valid. You, Karen, are a lighthouse in my ocean."

—A parent in Alaska

"This book has become required reading for my staff and a recommended reading for parents. Dr. Foli gives us all a lesson in persistence, patience, hope, and the importance of teamwork."

—Jacqueline Egli, Executive Director, PACE Brantley-Hall School, Longwood, Florida

Like Sound Through Water

A Mother's Journey Through
Auditory Processing Disorder

BY KAREN J. FOLI, PH.D.

FOREWORD BY EDWARD M. HALLOWELL, M.D.

ATRIA BOOKS

New York London Toronto Sydney Singapore

ATRIA BOOKS
1230 Avenue of the Americas
New York, NY 10020

ISBN: 0-7434-2198-1
        0-7434-2199-X (Pbk)

First Atria Books trade paperback edition July 2003

10 9 8 7 6 5 4 3 2 1

ATRIA BOOKS is a trademark of Simon & Schuster, Inc.

For information regarding special discounts for bulk purchases,
please contact Simon & Schuster Special Sales at 1-800-456-6798 or
business@simonandschuster.com

Manufactured in the United States of America

This book is dedicated to John, Ben, Peter, and Annie,
my heroes

Contents

Acknowledgments

THE EXISTENCE OF THIS BOOK IS DUE TO MANY PEOPLE'S BE-lief that the parents and children who struggle with auditory processing disorder (APD) deserve to understand what they are facing. With this belief, the following individuals, family, friends, and professionals extended to me their faith and encouragement:

Reno and Adele Foli, my parents, whose love for their three daughters showed me how to love my children. Leanne Malloy and Margaret Conway, my sisters and very special friends.

Jodie Rhodes, my agent, who believed there was a market for this book when many others did not. She used all her energies to do what an agent does best—shape the proposal, get it to the right people, and cheer me on during the writing process.

Tracy Behar, my editor, who supported this memoir, kept its integrity intact, and went above and beyond the call of duty to make sure it was the best it could be. She was the best first audience a writer could have.

Rebecca Leitman Veidlinger, my intellectual property attorney, who helped a novice to understand the business side of publishing.

My writing colleagues, whose invaluable feedback and enthusiasm helped me to see the text when I was too close to notice the blemishes: Sara Hoskinson Frommer, Rhonda Leah Rieseberg, Laura Kao, and Jeanne Myers. In memory of Margaret Anne Huffman, who will always inspire me with her humor, courage, and love of life.

The parents of APD children who shared their stories with candor, kindness, and out of love for their kids.

Teri James Bellis, Ph.D., whose commentary regarding scientific accuracy helped to clarify the complexities of APD.

Edward M. Hallowell, M.D., whose wonderful opening remarks situate the reader into the world of auditory processing disorder. He eloquently and insightfully describes the heart of this book, and I am forever grateful for his time and generosity.

And to John, my husband, whose unfaltering belief in our family has given me a future to look forward to.

To all of you, thank you.

Foreword

by Edward M. Hallowell, M.D.

IN THE FIELD OF WRITING ABOUT THE MIND AND BRAIN, books intended for a lay audience usually are either a) accurate in the information they contain but so boring and poorly written as to be unreadable, or b) well-written and moving but full of inaccuracies and/or strident polemics.

This book is neither.

No, this book is from heaven. This book is both carefully written and written from the heart. This book is both informative and gripping. This book both taught me and made me lay it down as I paused to gather my emotions before I could read on.

You are about to enter into the private world of a mother, her son, her husband, and her two other children. You are about to sail on the waters of their lives, waters that are colored differently on different days, as you will see. You are about to encounter a parent's worst fears, and you are about to sit next to one mom as she becomes a hero, right along with the rest of her true-to-life family.

Save an hour or two for savoring this book. Don't read this book merely as a resource book about auditory processing disorder (although it is the best such book I have ever read). Read this book as you would a novel, a story about discovery and disappointment, understanding and misunderstanding, learning and not learning, hope and despair, and love in the face of difficult times, love that never, never quits.

In this book you will see Karen and her husband, John, struggle to understand their first child, Ben. You will see them wince as they realize that Ben is not like every other child. You will see them wince again as professionals fail to get the point. You will feel their emotions as the child they love receives mistreatment purported to be help. You will see a mom, trying her best to work within an uncomprehending system of educators and healthcare professionals, refuse to give up on her son or relinquish her sense of who she knows her child truly to be.

There is a lonely, largely unrecognized crisis in many lives that this book brilliantly details. It is the crisis that results when you do not have correct understanding of your mind, or the mind of a person who is close to you, such as your child, or sibling, or parent, or spouse. Tens of millions of people in America today and hundreds of millions of people around the world lead lives full of wrenching, unnecessary pain simply because they have not yet found the correct understanding, or diagnosis, of the mind that they have. In this book, the elusive, correct diagnosis is auditory processing disorder, or APD. But what Karen Foli more generally recounts is not merely the journey toward the diagnosis of APD, but the twisting, turning road from a misunderstanding to an understanding of a mind, period.

Imagine if you had a child whose learning or behavior or emotions—or all three—caused your child and you and your family to suffer deeply every day. This is the case for many millions of children and families in America right now. And imagine if you, as the child's mother, had to go from misunderstanding to misunderstanding day in and day out, from "expert" to "expert," each with his or her own set of forms to fill out, tests to take, and jargon-filled explanations to listen to. Imagine if each time the expert missed the true nature of your child you had to choose between disagreeing and being told you were in denial, or agreeing and knowing you were not going to get the kind of help you so desperately needed. What would you do?

Science knows so much about the mind today. But we are using precious little of what is known. There are two major reasons for this. The most obvious reason is that so much is known now that no one, not even the experts in any given field, can keep up with it all. The subject of this book, APD, provides an excellent example. To provide proper diagnosis and treatment of APD, the expert needs the training and knowledge of child psychiatry, audiology, speech-language pathology, and occupational therapy. Rare is the clinician who combines the knowledge of all four; and even with a team that includes experts in these disciplines, the correct diagnosis may still get buried by the forces of rhetoric, status, or seniority in the clinic.

But a deeper reason for the nonuse of the knowledge we have about the brain is stigma. The fact is that most people are still afraid of diagnoses of the mind. It is acceptable to diagnose the kidney or the knee, but don't go near the mind! That is reserved for "crazy" people. This stigma perpetuates the forces of bias and ignorance, and denies the many millions of people who could get life-changing or life-saving help for depression or anxiety or a learning problem from ever getting it.

But Karen Foli would not allow her son Ben to be denied. In this book you will watch one woman, her heart nearly breaking, persist in loving her son, staying loyal to what she knew in her gut were his strengths, even as she rejected incomplete or incorrect explanations for what was going wrong in his efforts to learn and grow. You will watch one quiet, brave dad, who sees himself in his son, hang in there for him, helping his wife in his own special way, and helping his son with his own special love. You will see some professionals behave like bureaucratic fools, offering paperwork instead of empathy or knowledge; but you will also see some professionals come to the rescue, with knowledge and skill and caring hearts.

This book will teach you what you need to know about APD. But it will do so much more than that. It will give you hope, especially if you, or your child, or someone else close to you is struggling, not knowing exactly how to manage their behavior, learning, or emotions. This book will give you hope by showing you the example of one mother who at first had no idea what was going on, but with patience and determination finally found out. It will show you how one woman struggled to find a proper understanding of her child's mind, before too much damage was done. And she did. What an act of love. What a life-saving, determined act of love.

Some day, Ben, when you read this book, I am sure you will fill up with pride and admiration for this wonderful woman, Karen, who you are lucky enough to call Mom. Many millions of people will have learned and benefited from this book by then!

Introduction

A MOTHER ALWAYS KNOWS WHEN SOMETHING IS WRONG with her child. If it's a physical problem, the reaction is simple and swift. She takes the child to a doctor. But when the problem is mental or emotional, when the child is not developing as fast as he should, the situation is so overwhelming that denial sets in. The mother and father talk. Frequently, the father comforts the mother. He tells her she's worrying unnecessarily, that each child is different, that their child will develop at his or her own pace. That's what my husband told me and he should know. He's a board certified psychiatrist with special training in child and adolescent disorders. For that matter, I'm also a professional, a registered nurse who holds a master's degree in nursing and a doctorate in communications.

But I couldn't keep on denying what was in front of my eyes. My son, Ben, not only couldn't talk by the age of three, he couldn't comprehend the simplest things said to him. He wouldn't make eye contact. He was anxious, distracted, and although he reacted to noise, he often wouldn't turn when I spoke to him. Finally, I knew I had to act. I took him to a speech and hearing clinic. To those professionals and personal friends who were unfamiliar with Ben, questions surrounding mental retardation (a cognitive problem) and/or autism (a social and communication problem) arose from his presentation.

I have learned to never underestimate a mother's intuition. The people who had these questions about my son were highly respected professionals with all the modern diagnostic tools. They certainly should have been able to know what was wrong with Ben. But as I looked into my son's eyes, I knew they were missing something. I had no idea what the problem was. But I did know with certainty that he was not retarded, that he was not autistic, and so I set out on a journey. It is that journey I want to share with you, for although in a literal sense it is the specific journey of Ben and me, it is also the journey that every parent in the world takes to learn the truth and help his or her child.

CHAPTER ONE

A Healthy Baby?

I PUSHED ONE FINAL TIME AND FELT A TREMENDOUS RELEASE of pressure. Ben burst into the world, and I heard him gasp his first breath of air. A few seconds later, when he was nestled against my tummy and I counted ten fingers and ten toes, I felt an intense psychological relief that my baby was healthy. Healthy. That's what I believed.

"He looks good," my doctor proclaimed, her eyes excited above the blue surgical mask.

My husband, John, hovered above me and smiled.

"He's okay?" I asked.

"He's great."

And as my eyes met Ben's—a precious first connection—I thought so, too.

The pediatrician came into my hospital room the next morning and echoed the same opinion. Ben's Apgar scores had been high immediately after birth, meaning his circulation and respirations were good. Aside from his high bilirubin count, which caused his skin to have an orange/yellow tint or jaundiced appearance, he seemed fine. Ben was released with me to go home. The following three mornings, John and I brought Ben to the hospital for a blood test that checked his bilirubin count. It never exceeded the point that would have required Ben's hospitalization. We pushed fluids—formula, since my milk hadn't come in fast enough. Ben's body needed to cleanse itself of the bilirubin as soon as possible. The fourth day's blood draw showed a dramatic improvement in his levels. And again, I celebrated the health of my firstborn.

It had been a hard pregnancy. In the sixth month, I was hospitalized with hyperemesis, which meant I couldn't quit vomiting. But I figured it was well worth it. John and I wanted this child so much. We'd met later in life, after John had established a private practice in child psychiatry, and I'd turned in my dissertation toward my Ph.D. in communications. Our marriage took place a little over a year after our first date, and Ben arrived the following year. We didn't plan it that way. It just happened.

So when I had Ben at age thirty-two, I was more than ready for him. That's not to say I knew what I was doing. I was never one of those teenagers who baby-sat. Kids made me nervous. They were unpredictable, uncontrollable, and messy.

SIX MONTHS AFTER BEN'S BIRTH, JOHN AND I WERE READING in bed, enjoying a peaceful end to another busy day. Our baby was upstairs safe and asleep. Suddenly, long, incessant cries from the upstairs nursery broke the silence.

After a few minutes, I looked over at John. I always looked to him when I didn't know what to do. There's something in my husband that I'll never have. It's a quiet demeanor that at first meeting can come across as a weakness. But I knew better. It was a subtle strength that didn't need to advertise itself to the outside world. He kept it in reserve for those around him—especially for his patients and me.

"Just let him cry it out," John said. "Sometimes, babies just need to cry."

I forced myself to lie back and sighed. "Okay."

Silence. I didn't move, expecting any motion would somehow reach Ben on the floor above me. Maybe John was right. Ben was okay. He was just overtired. And there wasn't anything to do.

My eyes looked at the dresser where the nursery monitor sat. It was the type with bars of lights that responded to the noise in the room. The bars sat in their dark slots, waiting.

I blinked and saw an eruption of new cries. The bars seemed to blow off the side of the box. I shot a glance toward John. Although he was a specialist in children's development and mental health, I was a mother. At that instant, I was more knowledgeable. I threw off the covers, and my bare feet skimmed along the hardwood floors and up the stairs to Ben's bedroom.

I reached Ben's doorway, and he stopped for an instant when he saw me, clearly outraged at being put off for so long. I picked up his hot, strong body and curled him against me in the rocking chair. His nine-month sleeper barely fit him. Its white terrycloth stretched around his plump knees. My feet pushed to get the rhythm of the chair going.

"You're all right, sweetheart. My Benny." I pressed my lips against his moist head of light brown hair that was just beginning to bend in gentle waves. I was amazed at the softness of what was new to this world. He squirmed as if wanting to get down.

"No. Time to go na-na." I used the word from my childhood for sleep.

Ben turned his face toward me, and I watched him wrap tiny fingers around the button of my nightgown. I gently laid his head against my chest, hoping the rocking motion, a soft hum, and the closeness would help him to relax and go back to sleep.

He faced me again, as if expectant, waiting for me to tell him something. The August moon glowed throughout the room, bringing a calm to the night. The gentle light reflected off Ben's pug nose and round eyes, his mouth open and smiling. My perfect baby. An overwhelming sensation came over me.

"I'll always hear you, Ben. Listen for what you need."

His brown eyes, smaller versions of mine, peered at me.

I know he didn't understand the promise I was making to him that night. It was more than just a commitment of not leaving him alone in his crib. It was a pledge that for as long as I lived, I would do everything that I could to make sure he was okay. That I accepted my responsibility to prepare him for the world he would someday face without me. And I made this promise with a smile on my face, feeling his warm, even breath upon my arm as he slept. His legs curled against my abdomen, bent in a natural ball, as if reminding me that he'd spent less of his life outside than inside me.

What I didn't know that night was that my promise would be tested much sooner than I'd thought.

I LOVE TO READ. I LOVE TO WRITE BOOKS AND STORIES. IT followed that I would read to Ben. When Ben was about two and a half, we had a Winnie the Pooh "first-word" book that he liked to look at. John and I would sit with him and go over the words after his bath.

"Look, Ben, there is a bee. Bzzzzzz. Bee," I said and pointed.

Ben pointed and looked away.

"Here's Piglet. Piglet."

Ben sat there and made a soft utterance. "Ulg."

"Good Ben! Now here's Kanga and Roo."

Silence.

I leaned back, my eyes watching Ben. I'd read that book for weeks. Night after night. Sometimes, Ben would utter an intelligible word, but not consistently.

Later that evening, after Ben had gone to sleep, I said to John, "He's not getting it. He's not talking." I looked over at him, across the kitchen table. His blue eyes stared back gently, yet I could see some uneasiness. "I don't understand. He laughs, he's cuddly, but he's not talking."

"He will. I was a late talker."

"Is he okay?"

"He's fine." John rested his large, protective hand on mine. "He's a great little guy."

"I know he's a great little guy. I didn't say he wasn't. All I'm saying is that he's not talking, and he should be."

John remained silent, but I sensed that he was listening closely.

I poured more water into my glass and offered John some. "Ben's only saying a handful of words. Like 'doggie or boggie,' 'hi,' 'wow,' 'mama,' 'papa,' and 'all gone.' And the phrases that he says are run together so closely, you can hardly understand them." I paused, trying to think of an example. "Like, 'whereyougoin?' and 'whatisit?' He should be saying a lot more by now, right?"

"Kids develop at different rates." John put his hand over his glass, indicating he'd had enough to drink. "Let's give him a little more time. Don't worry. We'll keep working with him."

I wondered. And hoped. Maybe I started to deny that it was anything that couldn't be outgrown. After Ben was born, I'd decided not to go back to work. I'd spent the second decade of my adult life working and earning various degrees. I'd been a bedside nurse and an administrator, a healthcare consultant, taught in schools of nursing, and conducted research. It was time for a break, and I'd been advised that the preschool years went by too quickly. So, I'd kept Ben home with me. Now I was worried I'd deprived him of experiences such as preschool and playgroups that would have stimulated his language skills. My guilt had begun.

At the time, things seemed okay. By age one, Ben would play games with us, running back and forth as we caught him in our arms. He'd walked at nine months, strengthening his leg muscles on his husky frame. He'd also interact with us in a give and take of toys.

But his preverbal years—when he was one and two—were marked with gibberish, and he often didn't attempt sound or speech. When we spoke to him, he would often look at us in a puzzled way. If I put a tape in the stereo, he'd go to the speakers, trying to sense the vibrations. Yet he'd turn when his name was called, respond to affection and abrupt sounds in his environment, and when scolded, become tearful and sad.

And we'd added another child to our family, Peter, twenty-eight months younger than Ben. Our second son favored his father in fair coloring and blond hair. Ben looked like me with brown eyes, olive skin undertones, and curly hair. I started to tease John that Ben looked like me on the outside, but was like him on the inside. I'd heard that life grows exponentially when a second child is added, but we weren't prepared for what that really meant. Getting Peter's sleep cycle straightened out, well-child visits to the doctor, John's demanding professional life, and Ben's toddlership made for a busy pace at home.

Ben's compliant nature and sweet disposition diminished concerns over his lack of speech at well-child visits. At his two-year checkup, the doctor, John and I decided to take a "wait and see" approach to his speech development, to give Ben some more time. I'd also noticed Ben was a toe-walker when he first started to walk. The doctor would make offhanded mention of it, but I never pursued an explanation.

I knew next to nothing as far as early childhood development. John would explain it to me; he was my expert. He was the one who'd completed a fellowship in child and adolescent psychiatry, after his general psychiatry residency. He was the one who devoted long hours day after day to the assessment and treatment of children. No, my husband knew more than any pediatrician when it came to his own son's development. And I needed someone to explain what I was seeing in our three-year-old son.

"So what does toe-walking mean? Is it a big deal? Why does everyone keep mentioning it?" John and I were in the car, a rare night out—a Date Night. We were headed to a favorite restaurant.

"It's what they call a 'soft-neurological sign.' I wouldn't worry about it."

"What's that mean exactly?" I wondered if I wanted to know.

"It means," John explained in his soft, unassuming clinical voice, "that there may be something else going on with the child. It's not like a paralyzed arm, which would be a clear indication that something was severely wrong neurologically. This just means something *may* be going on. Not that something *is* going on. In Ben's case, I don't think there are any other deficits to be concerned about."

I took a breath. "I don't know. He doesn't play with his toys like I'd expect. Have you noticed? Take that box of sticks he keeps beside him. He even has one that he looks at a lot. And he stacks his toys in a nestlike pile, then examines them. Does he have any—I don't know—characteristics of an autistic child?"

"No," John answered immediately. "Autistic kids live in their own worlds. They don't have correct perceptions of their environment or the things in it. It's not Ben." John shifted his weight. "He's on target for his gross motor skills. He's affectionate. He likes to play with us. He knows the difference between something that's alive—like the dog—and something that's not." He steered the car into the parking lot of the restaurant.

"Have you seen that puzzle piece he likes to look at?" There was a Donald Duck puzzle that had large plastic pieces to it. Instead of trying to fit the pieces onto the board, Ben had become fascinated with one particular piece.

"He's all right. Look how he makes his needs known nonverbally."

I looked at John skeptically.

John continued, "He'll climb into his high chair when he's hungry. He points to things around him. He's even a bit on the dramatic side when he's trying to talk to us with his 'ohs' and 'wows.' And he loves to cuddle."

"Especially with you. It's like you two are glued together. I can't get him to sit still in my lap like you do." I caught a pleased look on John's face after my last comment and got out of the car, reaching to take his hand. There was an invisible bond between Ben and his father. Although I spent the majority of time with Ben, the two of them had this silent understanding of father and son.

We went inside and were greeted by the restaurant hostess. The local patrons as well as the tourists in the area favored the food there. Fried biscuits and apple butter were a famous side dish. We'd moved to the area a couple of years earlier—it was a much smaller community than Indianapolis. The dining room boasted a large hearth and limestone chimney that rose to the ceiling. It was a warm place, not just because of a generous fire going. It was a safe place.

John and I continued to talk about how late speech ran in his family. I recalled my mother-in-law telling me that one of her daughters was a late talker. One day, the little girl was looking at a jar of pickles and uttered, "pickles" clearly and loudly. That was that. Her talking began. I prayed to God that Ben would follow a similar pattern.

"I had a slow start with lots of things. In school, too, I was not what you'd consider a bright kid," John said after we placed our food order.

I took a sip of water, feeling puzzled and curious. "I didn't know you had such a rough time."

"Yeah, our housekeeper, who also watched us three kids, thought I was hard to manage. I remember being told to go outside a lot. And later, in grade school, I had a tutor and speech therapy. I think it was mostly for articulation."

But John's voice seemed light and matter-of-fact, like none of that history was very important, except to assure me that Ben, too, would be okay. We continued to eat and talk, reaching a consensus that Ben would be all right.

Peter was almost one and a really sweet baby. Slept well at night. Smiled all the time. Preverbal and verbal skills right on the mark with enough understandable words to make me comfortable. We just needed to start thinking about how to get that pacifier out of his mouth.

John had been asked to be a guest lecturer to the medical students. His topic: "Growth and Development."

"Why don't you videotape Peter? He's about as textbook as you can get. He's walking—although a bit unsteadily—reacts to us, and likes finger foods. I love it when he babbles and grins like he's telling us a big joke. Have the students guess how old he is."

John thought about it, but wasn't sure. My old teaching days kicked in, or perhaps my frustration at not teaching kicked in. "I think it'd be good for them to see it. Growth and development is so dry. Let them see Peter eating, cruising around, going up and down the stairs."

John started to nod. And I added, "We'll have the tape to keep—you don't use the video camera nearly enough."

It was left unspoken that we couldn't have taken a similar recording of Ben.

Our date night turned into a running dialogue of the boys. But something inside me fluttered and twittered. Deep, deep down. What was going on with Ben? When I was pregnant, I'd worried constantly about having a healthy baby. The nurses would catch me crying in bed while I was hospitalized, wondering what was wrong. The IV in my arm, filled with a cream-colored fluid, ached from the awkward position, but I didn't care because it meant my baby was getting nutrition. And if my baby was being fed, then he'd be all right. Now, I wondered what had happened. What had gone wrong? Was Ben going to catch up? Or did it all mean something more serious? I literally shook my head to try to forget those thoughts.

Everything would be okay, I thought as I reached for my third biscuit.

OUR HOME IN THE COUNTRY HAD EVERYTHING WE WANTED. A big, blue, salt-box shaped house, a creek, a pond, seventeen acres. Lots of space and lots of privacy. As Ben grew into his third year of life, I often thought of it as a sanctuary. A place where I could keep him safe, away from neighborhoods with kids who were quicker, sharper, and more able to tease him when he couldn't keep up. I envisioned losing him—he wouldn't even be able to say his name. I bought a harness, a yellow strap with Velcro closures, so I wouldn't lose him when I shopped.

On an early summer day, my parents came for a visit. My father, an elderly Italian man, was standing across from me as I washed the dishes. My hand knocked the green pot scrubber over the counter, and it fell to the other side of the kitchen island. Ben stood next to my father, and I said to Ben, "Pick that up for me, honey."

Ben looked at me, puzzled. His eye contact was good. I sensed he knew I was speaking to him. "Pick it up." I leaned over and tried to point to it.

Ben faced the floor, but didn't move. Then he stared at me again with a blank expression on his face. "Oh, dee."

My father's eyes caught mine. I could see the sadness in them, the pity for me, and the worry for Ben.

"Pick it up!" My voice rose, and my hands fisted under the cold soapy water. I waited and Ben stood immobile. I turned to my father. "Why doesn't he pick it up?"

"He doesn't understand you," my father said evenly. "He just doesn't understand." He stared at Ben, and then, finally, his old eyes turned away.

Ben's face grew serious. He had this ability to sense the emotional wattage in the air. I swallowed, desperately not wanting to cry, and thanked my dad as he handed me the pot scrubber.

AFTER THE INCIDENT IN FRONT OF MY PARENTS, I DECIDED TO try to engage Ben in more active play. I sat with him at the kitchen table, trying to entice him into coloring. He preferred his whale collection or his blankets around him. He loved to watch videos and would stare as the television screen played cartoons or Disney movies. But today, I was going to be a Good Mom. I was going to make this little guy of mine start to use his hands a bit more. After all, I had kept him home long enough. Preschool beckoned. He'd be ready to start this fall, in about five months. I just wasn't sure where.

I situated Ben at the table and held a crayon in my hand. I started to fill in the lines of the sailboat. "See Ben, fill in the bottom of the boat. I'm using a pretty shade of red."

I put a crayon into his hand. He ran the red crayon over the paper a couple of times, and let it fall out. I leaned over and tried it again. The crayon swirled around the paper and again, his hand dropped it. He murmured something unintelligible in his soft voice. Then he pointed with his finger dramatically, said, "Oh, wow!" and went into the living room.

The empty black-and-white pages of the coloring book closed spontaneously, and I put my head in my hands and started to sob. My fingers shook as I paged John.

When he answered, I yelled, "There's something wrong, John. You know there is. I know there is. He's not catching up. He's getting farther behind."

John's silence told me what I needed to know. Then he said, "I have faith in him."

"I'm getting him help. All right?"

"Of course."

"Have we waited too long?"

"No, I don't think so."

"I don't understand what's causing this."

"We'll figure it out."

"It's because I was so sick with him, isn't it?"

"No," he said.

"Was it the jaundice? We took him to the hospital every day. Why didn't they keep him?"

John's smooth, loving voice came across the line. "He'll be all right. He's got a lot going for him. He isn't autistic. Look at how much he loves us. And Peter. He's so gentle with Peter."

John had that way about him. My breathing got easier. I agreed with what he was saying. It was all true. John's strength reached out to me. Maybe it was because of all the pain and suffering he'd seen during his training at the children's hospital. I'm not sure. He didn't like to talk about it, but he'd told me about some of the dying children he'd tried to help. Whatever it was, he was able to ease my fears, provide the stability I needed. I trusted John.

"Are you all right? I'm worried about you. I'll call you later today, okay?" he said.

"I'm calling someone today."

"Okay."

"It'll be all right?"

"Yes," he said.

I hung up the phone, got the directory, and started looking for help. I found the number of a speech and hearing clinic at a local university. A major university. The woman listened in a careful, neutral way with "uh huhs" in all the right places. I told her about my nonverbal little boy. And added how cute he was. How well-behaved. How he made me laugh. Despite the crack in my voice, thick with stress, she didn't veer from her professionalism or invite me in emotionally.

She explained that they had a preschool designed for kids who had language problems. There was a morning and afternoon preschool program two days a week with individual therapy offered during that time. The therapy was delivered by the students and overseen by a faculty member.

"Morning is so much better for him," I said. "He still naps." I wanted to add that he was still a baby in so many ways, but didn't. I tried to focus.

"I'm not sure what the schedule is. Why don't you call me back in about four weeks and, in the meantime, I'll put him on the waiting list. There are usually cancellations. But I'll be able to tell you more then."

She went on to tell me that the program started in the fall, a couple of weeks after the semester started. Then they'd be making the graduate student assignments. But first, the testing. We needed to bring him in for a complete language evaluation. I had no idea what that meant.

"Has he been tested before?"

"No," I said.

"He's how old?"

"He turned three in March, and this is May . . ."

"Has he been enrolled in any preschool program?"

"No, I've kept him home with me. I have another son, an infant, and we live out in the country."

A long pause.

I licked my lips, and waited, sure she was ready to say what a shitty mother I was, and ask me why I had waited so long to get my kid checked out. Come on, I almost said. Let me have it. Say it.

Instead, she said, "Okay. Let me give you the clinic secretary, and she'll give you a time."

After a thank-you and a transfer, I made an appointment and hung up the phone, feeling a sense of reserved hope. And fear.

Then I felt something soft against my lower arm and looked up to see Ben's hand resting upon it. He cocked his head and laid it against me, trying to tell me it would all be okay. I laced my fingers through his hair and said, "My perfect baby."

CHAPTER TWO

The Evaluation

THE DAY OF TESTING CAME—WEDNESDAY, JUNE 7. A SUM-
mer day, when Ben's age shifted from "a little over three" to
"3.2," important terminology when kids are tested, at least to
those doing the testing. I'd arranged for Peter to be cared for by
our local sitter, Joanne, who watched kids out of her rustic home
atop one of the area's famous hills. Joanne's daughter had baby-sat
for us since Ben was six months old. Their generous natures had
been especially helpful. We didn't know many people in the area,
and Joanne had become like an extended family member, a large
part of my support system.

John waited in the car with Ben, and I took a shortcut through
the backyard to Joanne's house. I held onto Peter's hand, feeling
rushed, and carried his lunch. Not paying attention to where I
was stepping, I fell, twisting my ankle slightly in a shallow
drainage ditch. It hardly registered, even when I was back in the
car. I rubbed it, but my only thought was whether or not I'd dirt-
ied the skirt I was wearing. It seemed to make the extra weight
I'd gained, or failed to lose after the boys' births, even more apparent. I felt like a klutz, off-balance—inside and out—and I
kept thinking, somehow, whatever was going on with Ben was
my fault.

Or not.

Slowly, John's story had come out. Bit by bit over the past few months. But I wanted to hear it as a whole this time. Not in fragments. We always seemed to do our best talking while traveling in the car.

I turned to John after checking on Ben in his car seat. "So how'd you make it through medical school?"

"I did the exercises in the workbooks when the class had one. I understood the principles behind things. But I didn't read if I could help it. I was too slow, and it was too hard. Sometimes I'd read the textbook into a tape-recorder—without having to worry about understanding it—and then listen to the tape. I could comprehend better that way. I also would tape the lectures, if I could, then listen to them on tape." He shrugged his thick shoulders. "Studying was all I did. I studied night and day."

"Amazing."

"I read—maybe—a handful of books in college. But I had a 3.97 grade point average. My actual major was in chemistry. And I was good in physics. I scored one hundred percent on the physics final and left a half hour early. But I also had ulcers." He grinned as if embarrassed.

"I still don't understand how you got as far as you have."

"My mom helped me with my homework. And like I told you before, I was in speech therapy in my early grade school years."

"For articulation, right?"

"Articulation, mostly. So was my sister."

"What a family."

"My parents also tried a tutor. I remember crying during spelling because I couldn't get it. They put me in 'dumb-dumb' classes. I was told to use my right hand, although left was my preference. I was never formally tested, but I guess I would have been labeled dyslexic."

"You'd have been in special ed if you'd been in the system today."

"Probably."

"But somehow your brain kicked in?"

"Yeah."

"When? It was pretty late, wasn't it?"

"High school. I remember getting one of my first report cards and thinking they'd given it to the wrong person because it was full of As and Bs. I checked to make sure my name was on it. And there was a geometry teacher who believed in me. That made a big difference in how I thought of myself." He hesitated. "But it wasn't until high school when things started to change."

"Great." My flat voice fell into a whisper. Ben would start high school in ten years. A long time to wait and wonder and hope. I turned away and viewed the green trees and reflected that I should sense their beauty. With a mind too full, I merely noted that they looked like bushy stalks of broccoli along the twisting road. I heard John's voice beside me again.

"That's why I know Ben's going to be all right. I know what he's going through. I understand him. He reminds me so much of me." John glanced my way and then at the road. "And I turned out okay, didn't I?" He chuckled, as if expecting a tease from me.

"Sure," I said, feeling irritated at his complacent attitude, and started to bite a fingernail. But John's ability to verbalize as a child wasn't impaired like Ben's was. John had spoken at the correct point in his development. It seemed John loved his little boy to the point of missing something. But I had to admit his family was full of bright people. His mother was a retired physician who'd specialized in rehabilitative medicine. His father was retired from a long career at a university.

Sense. Logic. Cause and Effect. I desperately wanted to make sense of all this and I couldn't. I crossed my arms, and we rode in silence until we reached the testing site.

WE ARRIVED AT THE BUILDING ON CAMPUS WHERE WE WERE to meet Rita, a woman I'd never met but who I was told was in charge of testing kids prior to placement in the preschool program. Unfortunately, the building was under construction for a major remodeling project. It was a disaster. Particle board partitions cornered off certain areas, and I walked with John and Ben under plastic sheeting through which we could see black, bare wires and ceiling supports. It was like a cheap Halloween haunted house.

Ben's emotional radar was up and receiving lots of signals. This was not where he wanted to be. And I'm sure he picked up on my discomfort and apprehension. His gibberished verbal utterances told me he was anxious, his outstretched arms that he wanted to be carried. I did my best to hide what I was feeling and looked to John—probably unfairly—to keep the two of us together. To shut me up if I went on too long. To help Ben calm down. His mask, I must say, was better than mine.

We finally found the main office and were told to wait while they called Rita. I wrote a check for the testing fee. It was reduced, but the testing wasn't free. A number of broken toys and incomplete puzzles were available to keep Ben occupied. After a few minutes, a lady came into the room. Her voice was rich and warm, and she smiled in a welcoming way as introductions were made. Her gaze passed briefly over us and rested instead on Ben. He wore a striped blue-and-white shirt with an attached green hood. It reminded me of a sailor suit. He was one of the cutest little boys on earth.

Rita bent down, her long reddish-brown hair falling in front of her shoulders. She was in her mid- to late forties, and I started to breathe a little easier. I liked her. Ben made some eye contact with her and then came to be with John and me. Rita escorted us to the lower level room where the testing was to be done. We were surprised to see two young women in the room when we entered. Rita explained that these were her students, who would be participating in the testing of our son. That was when I first felt that the institution was there to serve students, not just clients. Education was as important as service, and I wondered if the two could be honored equally.

I tried to put Ben at ease, but he was on overload. Too many new faces. Too many new rooms. He turned away from those around him and sought out John and me to be held. They gave him some time to get used to the room, and that seemed to help. It was a fairly large room with long tables scattered throughout and a play area at one end. A one-way mirror took up almost one wall. But there were no real windows and the artificial light wasn't powerful enough to ward off the claustrophobic feel.

We signed the consent form and watched as they positioned the video camera on the tripod directly at Ben. John and I answered questions with one student, while another tried to engage Ben. John suspected he had had a reading disorder when he was a child—dyslexia—although he emphasized the diagnosis had never been verified by formal testing. He had been in remedial classes in elementary school. I informed them of the complications I'd experienced while pregnant—the hyperemesis. I was still vomiting straight into the ninth month of pregnancy. I told them about Ben's high bilirubin count immediately after birth. Ben's well-child checks were all unremarkable—he was in excellent physical health. No history of ear infections. He was always way above the norm in height and weight. He was a big little boy.

Ben still wanted to be near me, and I ended up holding him on my lap for much of the testing. At the time, I had no idea what tests they were using—just that they were testing his receptive language (what Ben could understand) and expressive language (what Ben could say). I'd brought crackers and some juice, and he sat at the table while they watched to make sure there was nothing wrong with his ability to swallow and manipulate his tongue. We told them that we felt his sense of humor and his affectionate nature indicated that he understood at the normal developmental age. What I wanted to say was, "He's normal. I know he's normal. I know what's inside him. If you look into his eyes, you'll see it, too."

"Marianne, why don't you show Ben this?" Rita passed the book, *The Three Little Pigs,* to her student, who then flipped to the first page. The women were on their knees facing Ben and me.

"Ben, point to the pig," Marianne said, looking quickly at Rita to see if that was right. She received a quick nod from the instructor, who had moved to a chair in the corner of the room.

Ben looked away and grunted. The student tried again. And then again. "Point to pig." Ben looked away anxiously and tried to move away.

I tried, leaning over him. "See the pig? Point to it." I waited. We didn't have this book at home. Why hadn't I bought this book? He'd have passed this test if I'd only bought this stupid book.

"The pig, Ben. Point to the pig," the student said again.

Ben crawled on my lap, burying his head in my chest.

"We have a Winnie the Pooh book at home," I said in such a soft voice that I'm sure no one heard me.

Rita stood up. "Stop. He's getting frustrated."

The student looked at me as if I should be able to make my son say or point to the pig. I glanced helplessly at John, who sat rigidly with a fixed neutral look on his face.

A few more tests ensued. Finally, Rita said, "That's all we're going to be able to do today, I think."

I got off my knees. "So is Ben pretty much like what you see when you evaluate kids with speech problems?" I brushed my skirt off and sat in a cold chair, my ankle hurting slightly. I was sure he was typical of what they saw. They probably saw a lot worse. They probably got kids referred from all over the state for evaluations.

Rita looked directly at me. "No. Ben has a significant delay. Very significant. Much more so than what we typically come across."

I don't recall much after that. Rita kept talking, and I kept nodding and pretending to understand. I couldn't let my guard down. Couldn't let them see how I felt inside. Not until I understood it myself.

Before we left, Rita took us to see the preschool room. We had to take an elevator up to the ground floor.

"Inowhyno," Ben anxiously uttered from inside the small moving cubicle.

I guessed he was seeking reassurance. "It's okay, Benny," I whispered into his ear.

After we got off the elevator, there were more construction droppings to walk around. I was carrying Ben, his arms tightly wound around my neck. He wouldn't let go even as I tried to show him the room.

"He's really attached to you, isn't he?" Rita said.

"Yes," I said with pride.

Her face became serious. "Well, we'll have to see if the preschool will work out. He's never been away from you?"

"No," I said flatly. "He hasn't." I walked around the room a bit, the toys and learning stations barely registering. I noticed another large one-way window/mirror along one wall. I heard her explain about the contexts of learning provided to children and the opportunities the children had to explore in the environment. Then her voice faded out completely.

I know I said good-bye and probably thanked her. I probably talked to Joanne when I picked Peter up. But I don't remember any of it.

ABOUT SIX WEEKS LATER, WE RECEIVED THE WRITTEN REPORT. It was my first experience of being alone and reading a test report that described my son as though he were one step above an amoeba, my first experience with how words were filtered and twisted sometimes. How sometimes the accuracy made me wince in pain. How this snapshot of my son became a document on file for people to read and retain as The Truth.

I paged John. I felt like I had my own personal crisis hotline with my private therapist at the other end. But he wasn't my therapist. He was the father of my children, and I needed my husband there with me. My legs carried me back and forth from the living room to the bedroom, the portable phone ready to be picked up when it rang.

John's work was always hectic; twelve- to fifteen-hour days were the norm. Healthcare—and mental health in particular—had started its spiral into managed care. Private practice was losing out fast. He was treating kids and adolescents mostly, but since becoming a father to Ben and Peter, he was having a harder time forgetting the faces. Like the kid who thought having lice in his hair was normal and didn't know what silverware was for and didn't everyone sleep on the floor with their dogs? Or the kids whose parents abused the Ritalin John would prescribe for their hyperactive children. Or the cases of abuse. Those were the worst. He'd report the perpetrators—moms, dads, significant others—but with a system already overwhelmed, not much usually happened.

John answered my page quickly. We had a code: I'd add a "900" to the end of our phone number if it was urgent. I used it sparingly, but five minutes before, I'd frantically punched the extra numbers in.

"We got Ben's report, and I don't understand it."

"What does it say?"

"All sorts of stuff about Ben's delays."

"I'm not worried about it."

"Don't you want to hear it?"

"Yes."

"They got our address wrong. Put us in the wrong city, for God's sake."

"They can fix that."

"They call me 'Mrs. Foli.' My mother is Mrs. Foli. Haven't they ever had anyone keep their own name after marriage?" Although I'd kept my name, Ben and Peter had John's last name, "Thompson."

"They can fix that."

"Okay, listen to this. 'The mother stated that she is very hesitant with Ben interacting with other children because of his size and she doesn't want him to hurt anyone.'"

"That's BS. Ben's got a gentle soul." John's extra beat of silence told me he was getting angry. "Why would they put that down?

That doesn't make any sense. We never said anything like that to them."

"I'm going to call them, don't you think?"

"Yes. Definitely."

"They also say he's delayed in gestures, play, language comprehension, and language expression. By months and years."

"They're wrong. I know he can't talk, but he's not like that," John said.

"Know what their number one recommendation is?"

"What?"

I took a breath. "'Ben should develop his ability to be separated from his parents and maintain composure to allow him to attend to learning task.' What the hell does that mean?"

"I don't know. Maybe they're afraid he wouldn't be able to be in the preschool. It's not important. We know our son better than anyone."

"They said Ben was 'noncompliant in his behaviors.'"

"He was just scared."

"I know. But that's not what it says. They're not going to add that the building looked like a damn dungeon." My voice cracked. "They say he's at the fifteen- to twenty-one-month age in expressive language. My God, he's almost forty months old."

"Honey. It doesn't matter what they say." John tried to calm me down, but I could tell he had to go soon. "I evaluate kids all the time, and I know they're wrong."

"Do you think this preschool will help him?"

"Of course. Let's go ahead with our original plan to put him there and see what happens."

"I think he'll be able to separate all right, don't you?"

"Yes, I do."

"You have to go, right?"

"Pretty soon."

I knew that meant, "yes." "Okay. Do you know when you'll be home?"

"I'm not sure. We're pretty busy. I have patients until five-thirty."

I hung up the phone and did my usual computation of John's arrival home. Allowing for time to finish his documentation, the commute home, and various calls from the staff, I'd probably see him around seven or eight. If I was lucky.

The report was still in my hand, and I started to read it more carefully. The assessment had been limited because of Ben's inability to separate. They hadn't been able to do a hearing test because of this. They couldn't even get a language sample—Ben couldn't talk enough. His gestures were those of a two-year-old. His play skills ranged from twenty-seven to thirty months, as did his language comprehension.

A one- to two-year delay in language expression.

I threw the report on the dresser in my bedroom. I didn't want to see it or think about it. But I couldn't sit still. The dishes needed to be washed. The whole house needed a good dusting, and I didn't even want to think about the bathrooms. But I needed contact with someone. I finally picked up the phone again and called my mom. I told her that Ben was pretty delayed in his speech, which we knew. Made light of it. This information wasn't new to us, really.

"Do you think he'll be all right?" I couldn't stop myself from asking. What a position to put her in—my mother, who'd raised three exceptionally bright girls with very modest means. My eldest sister held a doctorate in psychology and my middle sister was a certified public accountant. We grew up in a time before learning disabilities or special education or autism were discussed. The nuns, I was convinced, had scared us into learning.

So here I was asking an impossible question of this Italian woman who'd lived through the Depression, the death of her father at age seven, and a World War. Her husband, my father, was recuperating from triple coronary artery bypass surgery—open heart—done a few months ago. He was doing all right, but it'd taken a toll on the whole family. We'd been reminded of our mortalities, and my sisters and I had been reminded of how much we loved our parents.

I rephrased my question. "I think Ben's okay, don't you?" I needed my mom to tell me everything was going to be all right.

"Yes, I do." Her voice sounded like she wanted to believe it as much as I did.

"They thought he'd probably be okay for the preschool."

"That's good."

"He just needs to relax. I know he can do more than the tests say."

"Of course he can," she said firmly. "Ben's a bright boy. You can see it in his eyes. He'll talk when he's ready. You know what, Karen? I think all kids are a little weird. They're kids, for God's sake. They do odd stuff."

I laughed a little, letting go of some of the tension. We chatted a bit more. She asked about Peter, who was doing well. About John's job, which wasn't.

I thought about all the debt we'd been fighting since we'd been together. The divorce from John's first marriage had made several lawyers' bottom lines look good and, in the process, took his first private practice's financial cushion. Two years ago, we'd been left with legal fees, accountant fees, and tax liabilities, which had nearly suffocated us. More recently, John's new private practice hadn't worked out. Ethical differences with the for-profit hospital had made John seek a new position before we had had a chance to regroup financially. Old medical school loans were still being paid off. Now, he'd taken a large cut in pay to work at a mental health center as an employed physician, his second job change in three years. But at least it meant we didn't have to move again.

It also meant no more private practice. No more doing therapy with patients—according to managed care, that could be handled by the social workers and psychologists, or substituted with a pill. As a physician, John was now primarily a medication manager. An evaluator and consultant. No more autonomy and giving patients breaks on their bills or squeezing them into the schedule during a crisis. No more of that dream.

I didn't say any of that to my mom. She knew most of it already. But she listened to the latest round of events. About how John was making the transition to being an employee. She was a good listener. I asked about my sisters' kids—two preadolescent boys and a twelve-year-old girl. All exceptionally bright. All perfectly normal. As much as I loved those kids, I couldn't help but feel a twinge of envy. Why did my child have to be different? Struggle?

"They're fine," she said.

"How's Dad?"

"He's fine, too. It's slower on some days than others. Going to rehab is helping. I tell him not to push himself so hard, but you know how he is. And we worry about you guys."

"We're okay, Ma. I'd better let you go."

When I got off the phone, I couldn't shake the feeling that somehow I caused her more worry than my sisters ever had.

I sat down on the sofa and stared in front of me. I felt as if I were swimming in a vast ocean that I didn't know existed on earth. The water was dark purple, not blue. Not what I wanted or expected it to be when I was growing up. One that had tides that obeyed unknown laws, and I couldn't see any land on which to rest. I really wanted to get out of that water and just rest.

For the remainder of the day I took care of Peter and Ben, and ate, and watched the home shopping channels and marveled at how happy the television hosts seemed to be day after day. I started to know their names. And I waited for John to come home. That was all I could do.

I CALLED THE NEXT DAY AND VOICED MY CONCERNS ABOUT THE university report to Rita. Ben was not an aggressive child. He wouldn't hurt any child intentionally. He was extremely gentle with his baby brother. It wasn't that I was "very hesitant" to put him with other children. That's not what I'd meant. There weren't a lot of opportunities for play dates, but we had started to take Ben over to Joanne's occasionally, and he tolerated baby-sitters well.

I went on to my other points. How could they judge his play skills in a snapshot of three hours? What did "noncompliant behavior" mean? Oh, and the address and my name on the report were incorrect.

Rita was silent while I listed the discrepancies. Then she said that they had to go on what they assessed, but would watch the videotape of the assessment again. While noncommittal, she listened and gave me ample time to explain my objections.

I accepted this. I didn't have any choice.

About a month later, I received a second report. The report listed our correct address. I'd been elevated to Dr. Foli, and they'd added:

The mother stated that she is very hesitant with Ben interacting with children because of his size and she does not want him to hurt anyone; however, she was not indicating any aggressive behaviors.

Still not accurate, and I felt the incredible frustration at the anal retentiveness of the whole process. It made it sound like I was isolating him. Like I sat him in a corner all day while I ate bon-bons.

The cover letter apologized:

Following a complete review of the videotape and notes of Ben's assessment, we did find the need to make corrections as discussed in our phone conference.

The report pages seemed dry and sterile against my fingertips. I sighed and felt somewhat vindicated and pleased that Rita had listened, although portions of the test report still skewed my words. While the tests were supposedly neutral, the typed words of those giving the tests seemed to carry a final and unyielding power.

I CALLED A FEW WEEKS LATER TO CHECK ON THE STATUS OF Ben's enrollment into the preschool for language-delayed children. It was run through the university's speech and hearing clinic—the same place where the testing had been done—but different people coordinated the preschool. Ben had been accepted into the morning session that met twice a week. I was thrilled and grateful—a window of hope beckoned to me. This would fix him.

In August, we were asked to bring Ben to the school for a meeting with the preschool coordinator and preschool teacher prior to school starting in the fall. John and I were old pros at navigating the construction work, which seemed to be progressing slowly. I was calmer. No testing today. Just meet with a couple of people, chat, and no pressure.

After a brief wait, we were introduced to Cynthia and Beth, the university program coordinator and the preschool teacher. Cynthia was a tall, blond, attractive woman who spent time showing Ben around the room. He was calmer today and separated from me as he explored the colorful toys on the shelves. Beth, a pleasant-looking brunette, was responsible for filling in the gaps between the student assignments, and planning and implementing the curriculum. Beth presented us with a folder of forms, which included an emergency first-aid consent, and "consent for testing." I realized later that I wouldn't necessarily be notified when these tests were given to Ben or specifically which tests would be administered.

I signed everything they asked. For their protection and my son's, Ben couldn't be enrolled without the signed consents. If they'd wanted me to color a picture of a purple spotted elephant, I would have done it. Cynthia's voice caught my attention as I closed the folder.

"Big Bird, Ben." She held a Big Bird toy up for Ben to look at. "Can you say, 'Big Bird'?"

Ben looked away. I sprang from my seat. "He doesn't know who Big Bird is."

Her blue eyes surveyed me. She'd read the testing report. I was afraid she'd noticed the implication that I'd isolated him.

"It's just that," I explained, "we live in the country, and it's hard to get regular PBS reception. We get the Learning Channel from our satellite dish, and he enjoys that."

"Oh, I see. That's really helpful to know," she said, moving to a play telephone next. She picked it up and said, "Hello? Hello?"

Ben picked it up. "Hel."

"Good, Ben!" I said.

Cynthia nodded and made a note on her clipboard. She continued to show Ben around and then we were given a tour. Behind the large preschool room was a very small room where moms and dads could watch the kids during school. The window was big— about fifteen feet by four feet. A panorama of voyeuristic pleasure or academic study. A tiny counter extended from the wall and below that were about seven barstools to sit on. The room itself was dark, and we were advised we had to be quiet if we stayed to watch.

Of course, parents didn't have to stay. The children and students would begin the day with circle time, when everyone would sit on individual mats. Beth would then lead the group in songs followed by questions and answers about colors, numbers, and basic concepts. Then they would proceed with the day's activities. Snacks would be provided as well. During the course of the morning, the assigned student would take each child for a one-on-one session.

"Which is here," Cynthia said as she made her way down the hall. She showed us several rooms down a single corridor. "Each of the rooms has this box to turn the speaker on. You'll be able to hear what's going on that way." She turned a knob on a central box, positioned just below another large one-way window.

"Ben seems to be separating better this morning," she commented.

"Yes. He was a little scared the other day. And he's toilet-trained now, so that's an issue we won't have to deal with. He was trained over the summer."

"Great." Another note. "Do you have any questions?" she said as we walked back to the preschool room.

"How many children will you have?"

"Nine. There will be four students."

"Wow! Lots of individual attention."

"One more thing. There's another mom from your area who has a little boy starting in our program this fall. I didn't know if you'd want to car pool."

"That might work out." I sat down at a table in one of the kids' chairs and started to feel like a small child just wanting to go home.

"Let me get her permission to give you her number, and I'll call you."

"Okay. That'd be fine. Thanks for thinking of it." We chatted a bit more about the logistics of the program. The time it started, and that, in general, it followed the academic calendar.

"Anything else?" she asked in a professional voice.

"No, thank you very much." I stood up, and we left to go home with our son.

I TALKED FAST AND EXCITEDLY TO JOHN ON THE WAY TO PICK up Peter. Ben was content in the backseat with his McDonald's Happy Meal and toy, but I could see he was fatigued. Any outing, particularly to a new place, wore him out. Although I was hard-pressed to count a serving of fruit or vegetable in that meal, I would have written a letter of thanks to the company for inventing such fast, decent-tasting, kid-friendly food.

I kept checking on Ben; "You okay, Benny?"

He seemed very happy to be going home as his little pudgy fingers stuffed French fries into his mouth. "Wow. Oh, blag any ma." He pointed to his chicken nuggets.

Although I didn't understand him, I said, "I know, honey. We'll be home soon."

After a few minutes, I turned to check on Ben again. His little head was angled to the side of his car seat; his breathing was deep and even, and his eyes were closed in sleep.

The car seemed lighter—the tension gone from the morning's drive. My shoulders eased back in the seat. A hyperexhaustion filled me. But the day was turning out well. We'd found a preschool designed to deal with Ben's language problem. Six adults to nine kids, if you included Cynthia and Beth. An absolutely fantastic ratio. Plus private speech included in the preschool day. That would have to help him catch up. While the program wasn't free, it was reduced from what private speech therapy would have cost. And Cynthia was trying to put me in touch with another mom who lived in our county. Maybe she'd be willing to share the drive now and then. The first test report didn't matter. What mattered was that he was going to a first-rate program.

John's smile told me what was in his heart. "See, I told you it would be all right," he said.

"It's a start," I replied. At least I felt a direction. This was the best place for Ben. So what if it would take an hour's drive door to door, and I'd need to put Peter at Joanne's a couple of mornings a week. He was fifteen months old and doing well. It was all going to work out. I was betting that by the end of the year, Ben would be caught up, just like all those other late-talkers I'd heard about.

My voice became steadier, less breathless. "You don't think this could hurt him in any way, do you?"

"For heaven's sake, no," John said.

I laughed at my silliness. Yet, I thought back to a lecture given by one of my communications professors at the University of Illinois. She told us one of the basic questions asked by scholars was: Does discourse reflect reality or create a new reality? Can words and language form their own version of events, people, and life? I wondered about Ben's test report and how it veered from being totally accurate. Had a new reality been created for my son? And if so, how would that reality affect him and shape the interactions of those around him?

CHAPTER THREE

Through the
Looking Glass

DURING THE REMAINING HOT SUMMER DAYS, I VACILLATED
between thinking there was something incredibly wrong with
Ben and then deciding he just needed time: He was as normal as
they came. Just more time. After all, John came out of whatever
caused his delays. So would Ben. If the world would just leave us
alone for a bit, we could emerge in a few months, and no one
would be the wiser.

But when my eyes opened on the morning of Ben's first day of
school, I was instantly awake and alert. Ben had been officially
admitted into the Monday and Wednesday morning program.
My plan was to leave around eight A.M., drop Peter off at
Joanne's, get to the university preschool by nine, stay, and watch.
After preschool, I could grab some lunch with Ben, pick up Peter,
and be home by one. That was my schedule. My job.

It wasn't what I'd expected as my son's First Day of School.
This wasn't, after all, a regular school. He was there because
something was wrong. I held my breath and walked in, squeezing
Ben's hand. His hands always seemed warm and soft, and at the
same time, strong. They reminded me of John's hands.

After some initial hesitation, Ben didn't mind letting go of
me—the other kids and the lure of the colorful room filled with

smiling, pretty college students (all women) appealed to him. After a kiss and a wave from me, he went inside, and I dashed around the corner to the observation room. My eyes quickly found him. He seemed awkward, unsure of what to do, and I could see him swallowing, trying not to cry. I was sure I would at any second. He was such a big kid for his age. Not a good combination—large body and delayed speech. The expectations were already set higher than his chronological age. One student walked over and started to talk to him. She guided him around the room and finally got him situated for circle time.

I noticed Bridget, the woman Cynthia had spoken of as a possible car pool buddy. I introduced myself after matching the description Bridget had shared on the phone a couple of weeks ago. Today, she gave me a nervous smile. Her bright lavender coat contrasted with her black curly hair and clear pale skin. She was a petite woman, and I felt gigantic next to her.

I'd enjoyed our telephone conversation before the start of school. The parallels in our lives were astounding; Bridget was a nurse as well. Her son's name was Ben also (he was nine months younger than my son), and we had second-born sons the same age. She and her husband had married when they were in their thirties as John and I had.

Bridget and I shared the histories of our sons' developments tentatively at first, but I soon felt she was someone who was safe to talk to. I didn't have to worry about burdening her as I would a family member. I didn't have to worry about influencing a clinical person about Ben's delays. Although we never car pooled to the clinic, she would become an important friend to me for years to come.

My reflections of the past conversation dimmed as the immediate situation took over my thoughts. Cynthia sat on a stool nearest the door, her notebook in front of her with pen in hand, ready to take notes on her students and the children.

It was standing room only with moms. Generic moms. Big ones, little ones. Blondes. Brunettes. Short hair, long hair. Skirts, slacks. One was even in a wheelchair. About six of us in all. None of that mattered. We were a Collective Mom, void of individual properties, defined by the products of our wombs.

My past, how I used to define myself, was erased. I wasn't there as the Dr. Foli who had taught statistics to nursing students. Or as a long-term care consultant. Or as an academician ready to discuss media effects on health practices. Those were things of the past. I swallowed and extended my hand, feeling the cold, hard glass in front of me.

I was Mom, a stay-at-home mom (read: no professional activity) and specifically, Ben T's mom. Since there were two Bens, we were told they'd address our children with their last initials attached to their first names. Great. My son had a hard enough time with Ben. That extra sound would just make him more confused.

The other moms pointed to their sons and daughters, introducing them. The male children outnumbered the females by a ratio of seven to two. There was a small Korean boy, who I later learned had been adopted. He'd been brought to the States at around six months. There was a very pretty little blond girl whose history of fever, ear infections, and other difficulties left her partially deaf, Bridget's son, and other children like Ben whose speech was delayed by varying degrees.

Circle time began. Beth, the preschool teacher, sat in the twelve o'clock position with the kids scattered in a lopsided circle, some sitting on the young women's laps. The songs started. The "Wheels on the Bus" and "Itsy-Bitsy Spider" were sung mostly by the adults with a couple of kids slightly moving their mouths. I'd never heard those songs before, but I figured I should have. One student picked up Ben's hands and started to move them with the verses. He didn't seem to mind. But I could tell he was scared to death.

That was the moment I started to love/hate that window. I enjoyed seeing this firsthand view of my child's experiences. Knowing what he was experiencing would enable me to try to communicate with him afterward. I could refer to it and have an idea what the answers were supposed to be. I could let the students and Cynthia know why he would or would not know something and interpret what he might be trying to say.

But it felt like a zoo. On display were these children—my child—to be studied, measured, and researched. Ben didn't belong just to me anymore. For those two and a half hours, he was public property. It was voyeuristic. Each of us moms could see every mistake, every misstep taken. We could assess pretty quickly which children were the most delayed. The room seemed so small and closed, and I longed for a breath of fresh air, for light.

Cynthia left to go inside the preschool room. The Collective Mom was alone.

Another little boy, Keith, had been there last year and had been diagnosed with PDD—pervasive developmental disorder. John told me that was a diagnosis for overall delays, which included communication, social, and cognitive delays. I looked at the tall little boy with sandy brown hair. He seemed excited and wanted to be involved in what was going on. A little too excited, I thought, as he started to push. Beth told him to sit down.

Keith's mother, Maggie, said, "This program has really helped. But even before we enrolled him, we knew his memory was great. His dad showed him the pieces to a chess set one time. Just one time. Keith knocked the board over somehow, and he was able to put the pieces back in their original places and tell us—correctly—how each piece moved on the board." I'd noticed that touch of the Southern Indiana lilt at the end of her sentences. She smiled. The look in her brown eyes, though, didn't match the smile.

After a few "greats" and "wows" in response to Maggie, another mom chimed in. "Debbie has a hearing loss and wears hearing aids. They fitted them here for her. She came for individual speech sessions all last year." She introduced herself as Brenda, and I looked at her little girl, the pretty blonde whose long hair

managed to cover the two large hearing aids fitted into and behind her ears.

Someone asked tentatively if Debbie was born with a hearing
impairment.

"No. She had other problems and lots of ear infections when
she was a baby. We didn't know she had them. She had no symptoms of infection, and I took her to the doctor as soon as we knew.
She was even in the hospital once." Brenda was a young woman
with thick brown hair, neatly dressed, with a pretty face.

She shifted her two hundred-plus-pound frame on the stool
and continued slowly, "I asked about the preschool last year. They
said to wait until this year—they were still fooling with her hearing aids and doing hearing tests. They thought the social interaction would be good for her. She's our only child."

Maggie added, "Keith is an only child, too."

A husky woman spoke. She had frosted shoulder-length hair
and her voice was rough, skeptical, and rural. "David was here
last year, too. I think he's talking all right. But they said to bring
him back for another year."

We looked at her, waiting for an explanation. She shrugged her
shoulders. "You know how it is. They want me to keep him here
to see if he'll catch up for a regular classroom next year."

Silence. Then faces turned toward me. "That's my son, Ben.
The one in the green and blue sweatsuit." I smiled and pointed.
"He isn't talking as he should, but he's okay otherwise. He's so affectionate and sensitive. We have another son, Peter, who's a little
over a year old."

Someone mentioned they couldn't imagine having two kids.
Another mom introduced her child, and then Bridget pointed
out her Ben. And so on.

I looked for Ben again and recognized his back as he played
with one of the students. He seemed to be relaxing. He seemed to
be all right. The moms chatted a bit more, and then fell silent
again to watch the kids through the Looking Glass until it was
over, and we could go home.

* * *

OVER THE NEXT FEW MONTHS, BEN SEEMED TO MAKE progress, although excruciatingly slow progress. But John and I felt he was demonstrating new play activities, especially with his spaceships. And Ben had also added some new words, which included "bussie" for bus, "cheese" for cheeseburger, blankie, up, go, stay, Pooh, happy, and more question words like "where's?" and "what's this?". When he tried to talk, he had the appropriate inflections and feelings. But so much of it was still unintelligible. Or there were many, many times when he would ignore me. He'd look at me when I spoke, watch my mouth at times, and then turn away as if frustrated. Sometimes, I'd see such sadness in his face.

Peter liked going to Joanne's house. But he still clung to the pacifier, much to my embarrassment. And he'd experienced his first ear infection; luckily it had cleared up quickly. This little guy was emerging as a funny, ever-smiling, outgoing toddler. Although he walked a bit later than Ben, his development continued to be out of a textbook. He'd turn when his name was called and was able to enter into a dialogue of preverbal babbling in response to questions. He was able to follow basic one-step directions and appeared to his proud parents as a bright little boy.

Often, I'd feel these intense stabs of guilt because I didn't spend enough time with Peter. When I did, I was so tired. I seemed to be tired all the time. I longed for a clean desk, a piece of chalk, or a lab coat. Some research data to feed into a computer and have it spit back a statistic for me. To have something, a paycheck, a grade to show for this time in my life. Instead, I had a cluttered house and two children I felt I'd failed already.

I'd started to write fiction during Ben's naps as an infant. I'd continued, and it seemed like the only thing that kept me sane some days. It was my ticket to feeling control in my life. Characters could be murdered. Justice served every time. Plots fabricated at my whim. Along with the creative process came my naïve fantasies about becoming published and famous overnight. I'd show the Superwomen colleagues I'd left behind in the academic world that I could be a success, too. *Book One,* a medical suspense, was finished and I started to write short stories—backward from the usual progression. But it was just a matter of time before some lucky agent would discover me. Then John could quit his job, and with the advance money, I'd set up trusts for the kids. Ben would be taken care of no matter what. No matter what happened, if he had enough money, I thought, he and Peter would be okay.

I'D STARTED TO DROP BEN OFF AT JOANNE'S HOUSE ON FRIDAY mornings for more social time with other children. Cynthia said it was a good idea. John had adjusted to his job at the mental health center where he primarily treated the chronically mentally ill population. It was predictable, but he'd started to treat adults, which wasn't his first choice in psychiatry. He had to commute to three satellite clinics—two clinics were over an hour from our home. The long workdays continued. But we were in a groove, so to speak. The routine had been established.

Ben's assigned student, Carrie, seemed young to me. And so studentish. As a former teacher, I'd taught several students like her. The ones who were smart, read the textbooks, remembered what they needed to know, and didn't hesitate to look up what they didn't. They just hadn't learned about life yet or gained the compassion that goes along with it. Because of this, she kept strict professional boundaries. I felt objectified. Like a thing, an appendage to my son, who was her main object for study. Or maybe I just needed more than was realistic for this young student to give me.

I'd given Cynthia a copy of the words Ben could say at the beginning of the semester—about 40 words. Three months later, I typed up the expanded list of words Ben could now speak and gave Carrie and Cynthia a new copy. It was around 120 words. Way behind the 400- to 800-word vocabulary and 3- to 4-word sentences most three-year-olds are able to say. I noted any special meanings he attached to the words or any problems with articulation. He continued to say "boggy" more often than "doggy." They wouldn't let me count groups of words they called "frozen phrases," like "Where'd it go?" That was counted as one utterance.

The students were assigned projects that included presentations. About mid-semester, Cynthia announced to the Collective Mom that Susan, another student, would be giving an instructional talk on ways to improve our communication with our children.

The moms met in a small, cramped room. Susan was also a mother of a two-year-old boy. Because Susan helped to provide services to our children and because she'd never been defined by what her child couldn't do, she wasn't part of the Collective Mom. I felt a membership to a club that I wished didn't exist.

Susan began her presentation by passing around some handouts. "Okay, everyone have one?" She looked at each of us. She was in her early twenties, pretty with strawberry-blond hair. Her face always seemed to be bright and cheerful, her mouth in a perpetual smile. "Let's start then. On page one, you'll see some tips on communicating with your children. For example, shortened speech really helps get the meanings across to them. Instead of saying, 'Bobbie, go get me the pen on top of the table,' say, 'Get pen' and point to the top of the table. Nonverbal cueing really helps as well."

She hesitated and glanced at Cynthia. "Speaking slowly is also helpful."

I crossed my legs and stopped. Something clicked in my mind. Cynthia had mentioned that strategy to me earlier, and I'd tried it with Ben. When I spoke slower, not louder, to him, he seemed to understand much more. I didn't know why. I just knew it helped.

Susan had moved to page two and had included a page on signs of autism. I looked at the page, my heart beating a little faster.

Susan began to read off the page, "The signs include not being fearful of danger, inability to tolerate change . . ." She paused briefly.

I blinked, and my mind tried to connect these characteristics with my son. Ben hated change, but it was more out of anxiety of the unknown than a deeper problem.

She continued, "Delayed speech, difficulty in distinguishing living and nonliving things in the environment," her voice trailed away.

I let out the breath I'd been holding. Ben was late talking, but the other signs didn't fit at all. If I scolded him, his eyes would tear up. He could tell by the sound of my voice if I was really angry or not. He had a real sensitivity to others as well. I tried to keep listening to Susan, but I wanted to leave that tiny room and be somewhere else. Anywhere else, take my boy with me, and be left alone. But Susan wasn't finished.

With a photograph album in her hand, Susan told her captive audience how she used this with her son and how they talked about the pictures. How these contexts—pictures, events, and situations—encouraged his verbal skills to develop. I saw a little version of Susan on Grandpa's farm. In a toy car. With a doggie. She ended by stating the importance of reading to our children and then showed us various books as examples of good children's books to use with our kids. The pictures were a bit bigger and brighter than some other books I'd seen.

There had been few questions. One mother wanted to know if shortening the sentences would interfere with grammar later on. Cynthia added a few thoughts. Silence.

I sighed and tuned the rest of it out. If only it were that simple. There was this awful feeling that I could read and talk to Ben until I was hoarse, and it wouldn't get through. There was something missing. Ben's slow speech couldn't account for all his delays, but I knew they were not due to autism or because John and I hadn't given him enough contexts and stimulation. My question began to change from *why* Ben was delayed to *what* was causing it.

When Susan finished, I couldn't leave fast enough.

* * *

CARRIE MADE A HOME VISIT ON A CHILLY EARLY WINTER DAY. When I proudly showed her Ben's room with his various toys, books, and puzzles, she told me that I needed to keep it more orderly for him to be able to differentiate between the toys.

"Er, okay. Thank you for that tip," I said, feeling as if I were the student.

We went outside so Ben could play. He was comfortable with her now and hung by the rope ladder saying, "Hep, Hep."

Carrie smiled, "Well, we know what he's saying now, don't we?" She turned to Ben, "Help me! Help me!" This was to expand on the speech he did make, I was told.

Ben laughed and dropped off the ladder, making his way to a tree. There was an ant climbing up the tree, and Ben reached for it.

"Tree," Carrie said, brushing the bark with her hand. Then to me, "We need to get Ben to see the tree, not the bug climbing up the tree. The whole picture."

"Yes," I said, not understanding the why behind what she was saying.

Before I could ask, Carrie quizzed me again about my prenatal history and what Ben's typical day was like. She made notes for her report and then left. I never saw the paper she wrote from the visit, and I didn't ask to.

THE END OF SEMESTER CONFERENCE WAS IN DECEMBER. JOHN and I attended along with Beth, Cynthia, and Carrie. We all agreed that Ben had made good progress. Carrie read from her notes, "Ben met a lot of his goals. For example, he produced 61 intelligible, spontaneous utterances within a structured language activity. He produced 97 intelligible words during a structured play-based activity." She went on to outline the observations made about Ben throughout the semester. When she was finished, she looked up at John and me.

Unsure how to reply, I simply said, "We want to thank you for all your help this semester. We're very pleased with his progress."

Beth smoothed her brown hair behind her ear. "He's a delight. I've really enjoyed having him, and I think he's making real progress." She was the nonacademician there. Her role was to teach the kids. I liked how she saw Ben as a little boy first, and I trusted her impressions.

We talked about Ben's interest in whales and his whale collection and were invited to bring it in next semester.

"Will Ben keep Carrie another semester?" I asked.

"No. He'll have a new student," Cynthia answered.

I looked down and shifted my weight. "He'll miss you." I looked at Carrie. I had to admit, I'd gotten used to her. She did work hard with him during their one-on-one sessions, and she smiled at him more as the semester progressed.

"I'll be making out the student assignments over Christmas break." Cynthia went on to echo much of what had been said about Ben's progress. We left feeling warm and friendly. But I let out a breath I'd been holding, realizing how nervous and tense I'd become during those meetings. Because I knew during those meetings that I was the last person who had any real power to change their perceptions of my son.

THE WRITTEN REPORT FOLLOWED AFTER A WEEK OR SO AND was similar to the initial testing report we'd received in June. It surprised me a little and disturbed me a lot. To a certain extent, I balanced it with the positive feedback given in the face-to-face conference, but especially devastating were the findings of the initial assessments done at the beginning of the semester. Delays in all areas: speech, play, and receptive language.

However, the report reflected the progress he'd made. Progress measured in precise, minute, almost absurd ways, as if a yardstick could be used to measure my son's progress from the inside. Words and phrases created a Clinical Truth of Ben's progress— "more conducive to direct modeling and elicitation of language," and "increased use of communication strategies, such as eye contact and joint attention." The report mentioned that Ben's "self-stimulating" behaviors—it didn't specify what that meant—just that the behaviors became "infrequent, brief, and self-regulated," and that his eye contact had improved. He'd relaxed, I knew, as the environment became familiar.

But the flash of the first testing report and the innuendos and implications of a different reality—autism—presented itself again. I tossed the report on John's side of the bed for him to read that night.

JOHN CAME HOME AROUND SEVEN. I'M NOT SURE WHICH OF us was the more tired. As one of the few child and adolescent psychiatrists in the area, he was able to treat all age groups from children to adults. Because of this expertise, he'd driven all over the south central part of the state that week to the Center's satellite clinics. The boys were their usual active selves, and were all over him the minute he came through the door. I put the leftover dinner on the table, and he started to eat. We talked about his day, and then I mentioned the report.

"I don't need to read it."

"I beg your pardon?" I asked.

"I don't need them to tell me about my boy. I know him better than they do."

"But shouldn't you just look at it?"

His blue eyes looked into mine. "I don't need to."

I took a breath and let it out. Okay. I wouldn't argue with him for now. I wasn't sure if it was a mixture of fear, pride, or anger that kept him from looking at it. But I admired him for it. He believed in Ben, unconditionally. Yet, I would have to be the sole reader of this text. The emotions twisted inside me, confused.

Then I asked what seemed to be a daily, repeated refrain, "Is Ben going to be all right?"

"Yes." I could hear the impatience starting to creep into his answer.

"His progress is so slow." I pulled up a chair beside him.

"But he's making progress. That's the important thing. The preschool is helping him. They all said so in the meeting."

"It's your fault, you know." I looked at the floor. Suddenly, I felt something give inside me. Something that gained momentum that I'd stuffed inside myself, and knew I should have left there. "It's in your genes. This language thing."

Instead of getting mad, he replied in a low voice, "I know."

It cut into me, that tone of despair and guilt. How could I have said such a hurtful thing to him? John was always so kind to me. He was one of the kindest people I knew. He didn't deserve that. I swallowed, walked away, and let him finish his meal.

AFTER THE KIDS WERE IN BED, I ASKED THE SAME QUESTION as before, phrased a bit differently, "Is Ben going to be able to live independently when he grows up? Will he need to live in a group home?"

"What?" John's voice was angry, confused, and he looked as if I'd betrayed a trust.

I slipped on my nightgown and slid under the sheets. It was cold in the bedroom. The previous owners had put an addition onto the master bedroom—it allowed lots of light and lots of cold air in during the winter. I could feel the push of the frigid night air through the windows. "I just worry about him," I said sharply. "If it was up to you, we still wouldn't have intervened. You love him too much." More hurtful things. I hated myself and the anger escalated. And the fear.

I said my words carefully, enunciating them clearly. "Ben's delays are increasing. The gap between what he can do and what he should be able to do is getting bigger. His progress is too slow. Progress yes, but he's not closing the gap fast enough." I closed my eyes. My son was almost four. It seemed so ludicrous. At four years of age to be behind by so much.

John turned away from me and repositioned himself in bed. "He'll be fine."

"You always say that," I said in a thick voice. I felt I was being punished for trying to see what Ben's problems were, for recognizing that the water wasn't a normal color, but a deep dark purple ready to swallow us all up. "Don't you think I want to believe that? Do you think I want to think these awful things? You stick me out here in the boonies, and I have to drive an hour to get a can of dog food or a pair of jeans."

"Then we'll move. I'll do anything for you. You know that."

"We can't afford to. Realtor fees, moving costs. And besides, do you know how much work that'd be? Sure, watch two little kids and pack this huge household up. Which dogs do we give away? There's no way we can live in the city with four dogs. Do you know how trapped I feel? This job of yours—you drive to hither and dale every day."

"I'll do whatever it takes to make you happy. If it means moving, then we'll move."

"You love this place."

"But you don't."

"It's just so far away from everything. I don't know anyone besides Joanne and now, Bridget. I don't work, so I don't meet people. You don't work in the community—"

"I know. But you know I'd move if you wanted to."

"I hate it when you try to problem-solve with me. It just gets us off the track. All I want is for you to hear what I'm feeling."

I heard another sigh and felt his hand on mine. John couldn't give much more. He was exhausted.

John said slowly, "I'm trying. But that's what I do. You give me a problem and I try to give you solutions. I can't just feel like I'm doing nothing when there's a problem. I have to think of how to fix it."

"But that doesn't help."

"Just go to sleep."

I threw his hand off me and thought of the constant, daily inconveniences of country life, a life I once thought I wanted very much. "I have to drive to get the damn mail," I muttered.

We didn't finish talking about Ben or my fear. Just John's steadfast belief that his son would be all right. And his love for me, which I'd just met with anger. I heard John's deep breathing and knew he'd passed out from fatigue. I punched the remote control to the TV. God, I wish I had his faith. Pray. That's what I should do. But I'd been praying. Laying my hands on Ben's head at night, praying and hoping to God that He'd take this away from Ben and me. Make me ill instead, I begged.

But I felt no relief. Just a sick feeling inside. My painful secret surfaced. It was *my* fault, not John's. If I hadn't been so sick during the pregnancy. Able to control my vomiting. Not been so stressed. I wondered if it was the medicine the doctor had prescribed to help curb the nausea. I should have taken better care of myself. Of Ben.

Was there something wrong that couldn't ever be fixed? Was it that Ben just wasn't smart enough to talk? Or not able to, like an autistic child? Those thoughts flew in and out of my head with dreaded possibilities of a future I wasn't prepared to face. Thankfully, the images were too powerful to stay very long, and I glanced at John's sleeping frame to remind myself of what he believed about Ben.

I turned the silent TV off and started to fantasize about waking up in the morning with Ben greeting me, "What's for breakfast? I'm very hungry." Ben would smile, his two shallow dimples in his cheeks showing, and say to me, "I love you, Mommy." No trace of anxiety or fear in his eyes. We'd have the whole day to play at home. Or we could go to parks, malls, museums, and meet Dad for lunch. Peter could come with us instead of going to Joanne's, and I would have my boys all to myself. They'd just belong to John and me. No one else. No more reports, tests, or wondering. It would be so wonderful.

Finally, my mind wouldn't allow any more, and I fell asleep.

CHAPTER FOUR

Separation

THE CHRISTMAS BREAK LASTED SIX WEEKS. I WAS GRATEFUL to be able to stay at home with my little boys. Not to have to drive hours on end, to worry about icy roads or paying sitters or watching Ben through the Looking Glass. The countryside was filled with heavy white snow. If the snow fell four inches or more, our drive—a quarter-mile long—would become impassable, but I didn't care. I'd look out my kitchen window into the woods and sigh, wanting at times to never go out into the world again.

Being familiar now with the developmental issues facing Ben, I watched obsessively as he played or tried to speak. I thought back to Christmas at my parents' house the week before. My two sisters had brought their children—five grandkids in all—with mine being the youngest set.

Leanne's husband, Bill, was taking pictures. Ben, now with light brown curls like ribbons around his head, posed beside John.

"Smile on three," Bill said. "One. Two. Three."

The camera flashed.

Ben screamed in dramatic silliness to the bright light. And then laughed. He walked on his toes to where Bill was getting ready to take his next picture. Ben bent forward just before Bill pushed the button. Flash. Scream. Laugh.

"Benny, come here," I said, reaching for him. His soft cheek briefly melted into mine. Then he ran away to get into another picture.

I tried to look at Ben from an outsider's perspective. Toe-walker. Screams at flashes. Speech fairly unintelligible. I could guess what conclusions they would draw.

But the laughter. I knew he was acting like a little clown. An outsider wouldn't.

Today, the landscape outside my kitchen window stared back at me with its cold beauty, and my thoughts turned toward Peter. My guilt had now extended to the parenting of my second born, who was now eighteen months old. He'd had another ear infection that worried us, and we wondered if "tubes" might not be in his future. He was just a baby, and yet for most of his life, my attention had been drawn away from him. I wondered if he sensed this. Probably. Shitty Mother echoed again.

Yet I loved him so. Peter was funny. So funny. So alive. He had light blond hair, straight as a board, and slight buckteeth from his pacifier. One of my closest friends told me half jokingly that if you put Peter and me into a room with a bunch of other moms and their kids, no one would pick us as a mother and son pair. True, my dark curly hair and brown eyes were not genetically handed down to Peter, but I saw me inside him.

I noticed small differences between Peter and Ben. Things seemed to come from inside Ben, as opposed to responses to things around him. Not that he was in a world by himself. His emotions and what he tried to say, mixed with nonverbal cues like pointing, seemed to me entirely normal. It was just that he generated gibberish unrelated to what was said to him and appeared to be referencing things that he thought were interesting.

Peter, even though preverbal, was following simple directions and subtly responded more to us. He was active and curious. Loved the dogs. Would seek me out constantly and yet insist on being stubbornly independent. He had started into the "terrible two's" early and challenged us by being good for outside authority, but difficult when home. I was sure he was pissed-off at me.

John had been invited to apply for the medical director position and had just received word that he'd gotten the promotion. I was really proud of him. He'd made the transition out of private practice, brushed up on the treatment of the adult and geriatric populations, and was now demonstrating strong leadership skills. I just wished his hours weren't so long, and I weren't alone so much.

I'd prepared a letter to Cynthia and Beth, wanting to let them know about Ben's progress over the vacation. I also hoped that the new student would receive a copy and that it'd help familiarize her with Ben. His play skills had improved tremendously with favorite toys such as horse figures, dinosaurs, puzzles, airplanes, "spaceshippies," Thomas the Tank Engine movies, and of course, his whales. Ben could now make nonverbal sounds as well—for a choo-choo and animal toys. John's mother had given him a voice-activated stuffed dog for Christmas. Ben would speak into it, and it would repeat his words back to him. He now used pronouns occasionally and was beginning to use possessive forms of words. However, he was still very difficult to understand at times. I closed the letter by thanking them for all their help.

THE SECOND SEMESTER HAD JUST BEGUN, AND ONE DAY I found myself to be the only mother in the observation room. But I wasn't alone. Three other people in the room sat on the stools, occasionally writing in their spiral-bound notebooks. I pulled out a stool, sat down, and tried not to stare at them. I guessed they were other college students, but I was confused and felt they were trespassing. What right did they have to be there, watching the Collective Mom kids?

One plump woman looked at Ben through the Looking Glass and said, "Isn't he cute?" and pointed to her friend.

I grinned to myself, feeling proud of the curly-haired little boy who was mine. I watched Ben playing with some fish near the window.

Then I heard her say, "It's so sad." She bent down to make another note.

I turned to her sharply and started to say something. But I stopped and left the room. Left the building. Got into my car and drove away until it was time to pick up my son.

A COUPLE OF WEEKS LATER, I BROUGHT BEN TO SCHOOL ON A bitterly cold morning. The deep, penetrating chill of winter had arrived. But the preschool room looked alive with color and movement. The college students had really outdone themselves by making learning stations modeled after popular restaurants. One area was a grocery store with a pretend cash register. They had real Pizza Hut boxes, real McDonald's sandwich cartons, and other authentic supplies at stations where the children could pretend to order and pay for their food.

The kids were having a great time, picking up their favorite fast foods, and getting to take as much as they wanted of the pretend hamburgers and pizzas. The young women helped the kids go from station to station. It was a flurry of kid fun.

I crossed my arms and reminded myself of how fortunate we were to have this preschool available to us. Although we paid a fee every month, it was approximately a fourth of what we'd pay for preschool and individual speech services out in the community. All the pain-in-the-neck stuff didn't matter when I reflected upon it. I could put up with the Looking Glass and other quirks of this place. What mattered was that this was the best place for Ben.

ABOUT A WEEK LATER, BEN DEVELOPED AN EAR INFECTION— a rare occurrence for him. John had checked his ears with an otoscope, and we'd placed Ben on antibiotics. Ben didn't have a fever and had responded well to the first thirty hours of being on the medicine. I hated to miss even one morning of the program, and his energy level was back to normal, so I took him to school.

I'd settled into the observation room and had been chatting to Brenda, who had just joined Weight Watchers. I had grown to like her a lot. She was down to earth, and she and her daughter seemed to have a tender relationship touched with the typical battles of who was in charge. Brenda lived in a rural area as well and commuted to bring her daughter not only to the preschool program, but also for her hearing aid maintenance.

"You can have potato chips, just not the whole bag," she said grinning as she explained her new diet. "I figure I'm in my thirties, and I'm not going to have a chance to be pretty again. I'm going to get old, and if I lost the weight then, it wouldn't matter as much."

I nodded, trying to see the logic in it. Clearly, her motivation ran thin in the healthy lifestyle department.

"I've lost twenty pounds, but I was so fat, you can't tell any difference yet." Her eyes met mine, waiting.

"No." I shook my head vigorously. "I can see it in your face. I wish I had your willpower."

"Oh, believe me, it's not easy."

I told her about the writing I was doing. I was thinking about ideas for my second novel. Nothing published yet, but I kept the query letters to agents out there.

Brenda listened and nodded. "I think—"

Two women, whom I didn't recognize, popped their heads in the doorway and asked me to step out into the hall.

"Hi," said the first woman with rapid-fire speech and hurriedly introduced herself as an audiologist with the school. She just as quickly introduced the second woman, and I didn't catch the name, only that this was her student. "We tried to give Ben a hearing test today, and we noticed immediately that he has an ear infection."

"Yes, I—"

"We can't do a hearing test when a child has an ear infection."

"I know that."

"Did you know he had an infection?"

"Yes. His father, who is a physician," I said very clearly, "examined him and placed him on the appropriate medication." I waited.

"Oh. Okay." A giggle.

I shifted my weight. It was my turn. "I had no idea there would be a hearing test done on Ben today. No one told me." I paused for effect and looked the woman in the eye. "But I want this test done. He's not had a hearing test, and I think he needs to have one." I bit my lip. Because Ben reacted to abrupt noises, even to the point of being sensitive to sounds, we hadn't actively pursued a hearing test. I remembered his inability to have one done during the initial testing.

I spoke again, "Did he do okay when you started? I mean, was he able to follow directions?"

The audiologist waved her hand in the air. "Oh yeah. He did fine."

"That's good." I smiled. "I'd really like his hearing checked."

"We'll come back the next time he's in school." She started to walk away.

"He comes on Monday and Wednesday mornings," I added hurriedly as she was already halfway down the hall.

The instructor turned around, her white lab coat swirling around her. Then a pause as she checked her clipboard. "Okay, we'll work him in. Thanks."

They were gone. I was a little dazed by their manner of speaking and interacting. It felt so rushed and even confrontational. And I wondered how many times I had done the same thing as a nurse or teacher to a patient or student. I swallowed and went back in to discuss food with Brenda.

THE NEW SPECIAL FRIEND THAT CYNTHIA ASSIGNED TO BEN was a drop-dead beautiful coed. Aside from a clear, creamy complexion, she had long, thick brown hair and a bright disposition. When Kate smiled, I could see she was a good kid. But she was a kid. For three solid weeks, Ben worked with Kate on a Barney book that had all the imaginable combinations of rhymes of cat, bat, sat, mat, rat—every combination in the alphabet. Three weeks.

As I sat behind my private one-way window (a smaller version of the Looking Glass in the Collective Mom observation room) and watched his one-on-one sessions with Kate, I realized my son's case needed a skilled, experienced clinician. His problems were too serious to be a vehicle for teaching. He needed a pro.

But Kate did her best, and she was good to Ben, warmer than Carrie. Cynthia tried to pop in for at least part of the session, although she had several students going at the same time. One day, I brought in a few pieces of Ben's whale collection and his whale poster for one of their sessions. This collection meant a lot to John and me. These were toys that Ben had taken a sustained interest in. He knew the types of whales and could identify most of them.

I watched as Kate read from the poster and played with the whales, pretending they were fighting with one another. Ben imitated this model play. I saw Cynthia's tall form come into the room and kneel beside Kate and Ben. She held the poster and pointed to each whale, saying the name.

"Humpback," Cynthia said, pointing.

"Humpba," Ben said.

"Beluga."

Ben repeated, "Belug."

"Blue whale, Ben."

"Blue whale."

Cynthia paused, glancing over the poster. "Northwest narwhal whale." She started to laugh, assuming there was no way that he could say it. And there wasn't. I knew as a former clinician how humor could replace stressful situations. How it could alleviate a tense moment. The chuckle seemed to repeat in my mind, louder each time. I stood there alone in the darkened room, and something torturous stabbed me deep inside.

BETH PROVIDED SNACKS TO THE KIDS DURING THE PRE-school morning. On a day with just a hint of spring in the air, she made English muffin pizzas for the kids. Ben loved pizza. And he loved to eat.

The Collective Mom was in the Looking Glass room, and Cynthia said, "Can't beat that, can you? Therapy for your kids and lunch to boot. Don't even have to worry about feeding them when you get home."

A few moms nodded and kept silent. I felt my hands perspire and my fist clench and unclench. I let out the breath I was holding and told myself to relax. Cynthia left to go into the preschool room, and we watched the kids being served. The rule was that the child was supposed to ask for his food.

Ben had already wolfed down two pizzas and said, "Mo."

"More what, Ben?" Beth asked.

"Mo." He held his plate up in the air.

"More P-I-Z-Z-A," she said, slowly.

"Mo."

Other children were served. I could see Ben's confusion at why he wasn't getting more. I shifted my weight and closed my eyes, wave upon wave of anger hitting me. He half-stood, his plate held in front of him, waiting.

Just give him the f—— pizza, I thought. I opened my eyes. But Ben wasn't at the table anymore. I couldn't tell if he'd left the table before or after getting another serving.

TOWARD THE END OF FEBRUARY, I WROTE ANOTHER LETTER to Cynthia and Beth regarding some of my concerns about snack time (prompted by the pizza day), and I also thought he needed help focusing during free playtime where the kids could do what they wanted. Ben seemed to wander throughout the room at times. I questioned if the other available toys besides whales would be a good idea. It seemed that with his expanding interests, other objects could be used. Cynthia took it gracefully and thanked me. That day, she and I were alone in the observation room. I took the opportunity to talk to her privately.

"Who are the students I sometimes see in this room? They weren't here last semester."

"They're beginning students assigned to observe."

"Sometimes they make comments about the kids."

She looked at me and narrowed her eyes, as if pondering a question. "I see. I'll talk to their professor. They have permission to be in here."

"Okay." I looked out into the room, not really focusing on anything. I could tell the subject was closed.

THE END OF THE SEMESTER APPROACHED. IT WAS THE MIDDLE of April, and the preschool was scheduled to end a few weeks before the academic semester. Cynthia usually told the Collective Mom a few days before of any schedule change, and she'd just finished taping a sign-up sheet on the observation room door that read: "Final Conferences." I signed Ben up, trying to think which times were best for John.

The end of the semester also meant saying "good-bye" to the Collective Mom. I saw Maggie, Keith's mother, and started to talk to her.

"So, I guess I'll see you next year."

"I'm not sure. The doctor said the profile of PDD didn't fit Keith now. His development is on track. He's going to be just fine." The last two words were said slowly, deliberately, and happily.

"That's great!" I said, thinking of the tall boy who could remember the pieces to a chess set after being shown one time.

Maggie's smooth face no longer looked tight and constrained. "He said Keith didn't have PDD after all."

A few other moms were around and echoed their happiness for her. I kept silent and listened to the general chatter of the Collective Mom. Maggie started to talk about how she hadn't worked outside the home due to Keith's difficulties. I mentioned Peter and how I'd decided to stay at home.

"I think we'll just stick with one child."

"Oh," I said, thinking she looked younger than I.

"We thought about another one, but after Keith's problems . . ." She looked directly at me. "I don't think I could go through it again."

Before I could say anything, she continued.

"We thought about it and were going to start trying, but then Keith started to have problems, and we just couldn't see having a baby and dealing with all that." There was sadness to her voice. And regret?

"Yeah, I can see how you'd feel." I shut my mouth and wondered what her decision would have been if she'd known the doctor had misdiagnosed her child. I wondered what Maggie must feel. Relief. But surely some anger as well. Her face—her eyes— told me the fear she'd lived with during Keith's early life had frozen her against the idea of another. Too much risk.

The kids started to gather by the door of the preschool, getting ready to meet their mommies. I waited my turn outside the door of the observation room. My mind wandered.

I had helped to run John's office during our early years together, when he was in private practice. I remembered one evening—he saw patients until 8:30 P.M. three nights a week. A patient had called and needed to talk to him. It sounded urgent, so I had no choice but to interrupt his session with a young child of about four or five. After knocking, I slowly opened the door and looked over at his desk. It was empty. There on the floor were John and this little boy playing Lego blocks. I explained he was needed on the phone, and he apologized to the little guy and took the call.

Later, after the session, I asked John, "What's wrong with that little boy?"

"I don't know yet."

"You don't know?"

"No. I need to spend some more time with him. It could be a couple of different things, but I don't want to make a diagnosis until I'm sure."

After another session, John had reached a diagnosis of Anxiety Disorder. I thought about that for a long time. My husband was secure enough to admit he didn't know, but would, given more time and information. That luxury—extra time with a patient, a child—was a thing of the past. Now, managed care reviewers allowed less time for evaluations. But what of the Maggies and the Keiths? What did that lack of time mean to families?

One of the Collective Moms accidentally nudged me from behind and the memory faded.

Maggie smiled at me, wished me the best, and walked out.

I saw Brenda in front of me. She'd continued her weight loss and was up to almost forty pounds. She looked great, and I told her so.

"I exercise all the time," she said, as if this was not a positive thing.

"Will you bring your daughter back next year?"

She inhaled, "Probably."

We chatted a bit more about how her husband had handled her weight loss and laughed, after she admitted he was jealous of her getting some attention from other men. Bridget nodded to me. She was a few moms ahead of me and greeted her son, who'd just popped out of the preschool room. Although we usually had our own errands to run and didn't car pool, we'd become friends and had eaten breakfast together during a couple of the preschool mornings. She and I confided freely about our sons' difficulties, knowing the other one understood how much small successes meant. We cheered each other on, listened to frustrations, and in an unspoken way, knew how our lives had been changed by our sons. I realized how much I would miss the Collective Mom.

JOHN SAID THE TIME FOR THE CONFERENCE WORKED FOR him, and a couple of weeks later, the day of Ben's final evaluation arrived. We'd driven separately—John needed to get back to work—and I'd left the kids at Joanne's. Although these meetings always made me nervous, I didn't think there was anything in particular to be worried about. In my mind, Ben had improved, and I thought Beth and Cynthia shared that view.

It started much the same way as the evaluation before Christmas had.

Kate, Beth, and Cynthia sat together, and John and I finished out a semicircle. We met in Cynthia's office where there was privacy.

"Why don't you tell us your impression of Ben at this point?" Cynthia said.

I jumped in. "I think he's doing great. He's talking better, although as you know, it's difficult to understand him at times."

"He's playing with a lot of different toys." John's smooth voice came from beside me. "He loves his whales."

Kate nodded. "We played with those a lot this year. And we worked on his articulation with the Barney rhyming book." A gorgeous smile.

Cynthia cleared her throat. "We did do some testing with Ben to assess his speech and language abilities. In his Peabody Picture Vocabulary Test–Revised, Ben scored in the 'extremely low' range with a score of 43. The CELF-P test—it stands for the 'Clinical Evaluation of Language Fundamentals–Preschool'—was attempted, but due to Ben's inability to perform, we were unable to administer the entire test."

I stared ahead. What was going on? Last semester, the report was based on observational data only. No formal testing had been done. I'd missed some of the one-on-one sessions with Kate. Cynthia must have given him the tests then. I was probably running some stupid errand or picking up supplies. They never told me they were going to do these tests, but hadn't I signed the consent for testing?

"What does the Peabody measure?" I finally asked.

"Vocabulary comprehension. It is a commonly used test of receptive vocabulary with well-documented validity."

"But he has trouble verbalizing—"

"This test takes that into account. The child is asked to point to the response, not say it." Cynthia's voice was different. Low and smaller. Her blond head was bent above the paper. Beth and Kate solemnly listened to her brief summary of results.

Silence.

Cynthia continued. "He almost got some right. He was really close on a few. For example, I showed him a picture of a web and he said, 'spider.' But I can't count that. Then he said, 'towel' for a picture of the American flag. So he was close on some."

"I see." I crossed my legs. Why did Cynthia do the testing? She hardly interacted with Ben. Perhaps that's the way it was supposed to be. These were the experts. I didn't know this stuff. Stupid. Stupid. I should have stayed for the entire time.

I kicked into cover-up mode. Keep that smile. Nod. Pretend to understand. Pretend that what they're saying about your kid is neutral, scientific, factual.

John seemed stunned. It had been read so quickly. Neither of us knew what to say.

"I'd like to read my summary of Ben from the semester." Beth held her paper in her hand as she read: "Ben has made great improvement in his interactions with others. He initiates conversation with adults and is beginning to try to communicate with his peers in the classroom. He has a wonderful sense of humor. He continues to enjoy helping and pleasing others and is willing to take turns and share. He continues to be interested in his favorite subjects (whales and fish), but has broadened his topics to include other things. He needs to continue working on colors, counting, shapes, and writing his name. He enjoys singing and saying rhymes and finger plays. His vocabulary has expanded a great deal." She lifted her head up after reading.

"Thank you." I said, totally confused. "He's able to interact more with the children, don't you think?"

Cynthia said, "Yes, but you can refer to the report as far as his needs." She nodded to the report we'd been handed a few minutes before and inhaled before saying, "Some autistic kids have thought processes that—"

"He's not autistic," John blurted out. His face was red, and he wore a half-smile I knew well. A smile created from anger and frustration.

My heart seemed to skip beats, thinking back to the student presentation last semester on signs of autism. I glanced at John, then to Cynthia.

All three women looked away from us.

"He's not," I said.

Silence. With my eyes now averted, a struggle within me made me start and stop, wanting to ask more questions, yet afraid. Afraid of not showing deference to my husband and being disloyal to my child, that my comments might hurt Ben somehow. Afraid of the power I perceived this institution to hold. And at a loss to know the right questions to ask.

Cynthia spoke, "You'd mentioned setting up some private speech therapy for Ben over the summer. I need to check with Dr. Hartman to see which students will be available this summer."

"That'd be fine," I murmured. I remembered Dr. Hartman was the big cheese at the clinic. I'd never seen her.

"I'll call you next week and let you know for sure."

"I'd like to have Ben get some speech therapy over the summer. I'd appreciate whatever you can set up."

We murmured our thanks and wished Kate the best with her future plans. Then John and I left the room. My legs felt stiff, and I moved like a robot to the car. I should understand. What had just happened? John. John could tell me what it all meant.

We reached my car. I turned away from the clinic, fearful of someone seeing my tears that now fell. The questions exploded.

"What are they saying? What does that test mean? Are they saying he's retarded?"

"He's not."

"But what are they trying to tell us?"

"I don't know. They're only qualified to diagnose speech and language issues."

"I know that. But what do those tests mean? Is he mentally handicapped?"

"No!"

"He isn't comprehending. Why can't he understand? Do the scores say he's retarded?"

John stood there. The color of his blue eyes matched the overcast day. "I don't know. But the tests don't mean anything. They're wrong. I know my boy. He's not stupid. And he's not autistic. He just can't talk. But he will. I know he will."

I desperately wanted to believe him and clung to his arm.

He shook his head. "I feel like they don't give me any credit for what I know. I evaluate kids for the diagnoses they're inferring. Ben isn't those things. They're way out of line."

I drew his arm closer to me.

He swallowed and for a moment, his sadness engulfed me. "I know where Ben's coming from. I can't explain it."

We stood there for a moment, helplessness washing over me.

"Go on. You need to go to work or you'll be even more behind. I need you to get home as soon as possible. Go," I said, trying to block the tears.

He kissed me and told me it would be all right. I could see the lingering anger in his eyes. The hurt as well. I envied him that he'd have something to take his mind off all this. I dreaded being alone when I got home.

I drove back to the small town where we lived and pulled into Joanne's gravel road. Her house seemed a welcome picture in simplicity.

I got out of the car. I told myself not to cry. I wasn't a public person. Displays of emotion were kept in the home. But when I saw Joanne coming out of the house with my two little boys, I burst into tears.

I couldn't speak for a moment. I tried to catch my breath and uttered, "They think Ben's retarded."

"That's bullshit," Joanne said. She was a pretty woman in her early fifties with dark eyes and long black hair. "He's the smartest boy here. All the other kids want to do what he does. He catches on really fast to new things. They don't know what they're talking about. I've watched kids for over twenty years, and I know he's a smart kid."

I looked her in the eye. She didn't blink. "Thanks. They didn't come right out and say it, but the test scores are so low."

"Those tests don't mean anything. I know."

I swallowed, wiped my cheeks off, and exhaled. God, I wanted to believe her. She didn't study Ben. She took care of him and saw him first as a child, second as a child who couldn't talk.

"Come on, guys." I took my boys' hands and loaded them into the car. Their subdued manners and curious stares at my now red nose and puffy eyes were met with a weak smile from me. "It's okay. Mommy is just a little sad." I finished buckling Pete into his car seat, and Ben into his booster strap. Then we went home.

After getting the kids a snack and putting a movie in the VCR for them to watch, I turned to the report:

Goldman-Fristoe Test of Articulation: A phonetic inventory was given. Ben used lots of substitutions for the correct phonemes, such as "siz" for "scissors" and "frok" for "frog." He had final sound deletions, such as "penci" for "pencil." But even with the report in front of me, I couldn't understand the results. Sentences like "Ben's substitutions were inconsistent, but he most frequently substituted voiceless stops for all other sounds across word position" left me clueless as to what was concluded.

Play skills at sixteen to twenty-two months of age as measured by the Development of Pretend/Symbolic Play. I laid the paper down. They never mentioned this. I wrote the letter after Christmas break that described the toys Ben had started to play with. None of it mattered. None of it.

Clinical Evaluation of Language Fundamentals–Preschool or CELF-P: No score possible, as Ben was able to do only two, one expressive and one receptive, of the six subtests. No scores could be reported since the entire test couldn't be given. What little he was able to do, Ben performed better on the expressive subtest, able to say "making drink" when shown a man pouring a drink, and "sock/shoe" when shown a picture of a sock. He called a picture of a web, a "spider," as Cynthia had said, and a picture of a turkey, a "bird." Receptively, he couldn't respond to the specific one-level oral directions.

Peabody Picture Vocabulary Test–Revised, the test of vocabulary comprehension, where Ben was asked to "Point to_____" after being shown four pictures: Ben scored in the "Extremely Low" range. Again, the report seemed abstract and hard to decipher. His percentile rank was –1. Was that possible?

And no results from any hearing test.

Numbness. I couldn't feel anymore at that particular moment, but went to seek my boys out. I walked into the living room and felt their hands. Warm and soft and new. I kissed their cheeks and felt a little spit slide out from under Peter's pacifier. I sat down and watched the Disney movie I'd seen a dozen times, and tried to gain strength from their presence.

I TALKED TO BRIDGET A COUPLE OF DAYS LATER, EACH OF US giving the highlights of the test reports. Her son had done average on the Peabody Picture Vocabulary test and overall, better than my Ben on expression and receptive abilities. Again, we commiserated about the preschool, the test results and inferences that had been made. But I was beginning to feel that although our sons' difficulties surrounded speech, each boy presented unique challenges. Bridget's conference had been after mine, and she told me individual speech sessions were going to be set up with her son for the summer.

"Cynthia told me she'd have to check," I said.

"She told me they could do it."

"Why did she say she'd have to check?"

"I don't know, Karen. All I know is that they said it could be arranged."

I hung up after a bit and a steady, strong anger came over me.

* * *

JOHN HAD CONSULTED WITH SOME OF THE PSYCHOLOGISTS AT work about the concept of a negative rank score. They all agreed it wasn't conceptually accurate. We'd read Ben's report again and again. The tests scores' power played out on the page. Inescapable. Objective. Proof.

And yet, there were discrepancies we could not let go—for Ben's sake. We decided to write a letter to Dr. Hartman.

John and I sat talking at the kitchen table while the kids slept upstairs. The conference had been five days earlier. His eyes were swollen with fatigue, and his back was stooped. I felt achy and old, and I vacillated between feeling so very tired inside and almost incoherent with anger at the clinic. There was now a common enemy. John and I were united, fighting for the benefit of our son. Our commitment to each other solidified as our fury over the report escalated.

"Rob said there was no way a −1 rank is theoretically sound. He said it's absurd." John referred to his colleague at the hospital, a trained psychologist with years of experience.

"What gets me is the fact that we were invited to give our view of Ben and no one contradicted us. No one said a word about what we reported about his play skills. Sixteen to twenty-two months, I mean, come on." I paused. "Do you want me to read the letter?" John still liked hearing words as opposed to reading them, particularly when he was tired.

After he nodded, I began. "We are writing this letter to bring to your attention the serious concerns we are having regarding the preschool program."

John closed his eyes, and I continued reading the letter. About how we'd received nothing but positive feedback from Cynthia throughout the semester. She told us Ben was doing "wonderfully." We were assured individual speech sessions over the summer could be set up. Now it seemed we'd been misled. We questioned the −1 rank on the Peabody test as a theoretical concept, and demanded the original Peabody data be shown to us and the results struck from his final report. We questioned why Ben had never received a follow-up hearing test, which we'd specifically requested. We questioned why Beth's report differed so much from the one submitted by Cynthia. We questioned why a person who'd spent the least amount of time with Ben, would do such important testing.

We rejected their assessment of Ben's play skills at the sixteen- to twenty-two-month level as "inaccurate and misleading." We revoked "all prior consents for treatment, dissemination of test scores, and other related information collected during the course of our son's treatment."

We wrote about how the Collective Mom was informed at the last minute of schedule changes and how we believed that the philosophy of the school—education—seemed to take priority over any real commitment to service. We ended the letter by saying that, "lives are affected by these services and reports."

John nodded. "Good. That's good."

I smiled; I'd written the letter willingly. Almost with pleasure. It was the angriest letter I'd ever written in my life, and I sent it certified mail the next day.

TWO WEEKS LATER, WE GOT OUR RESPONSE. THE ORIGINAL Peabody test data were enclosed. A revised "Summary of Progress" was included. Dr. Hartman also attached detailed information regarding how the play skills were assessed. She pointed out that Cynthia was trained to administer the tests and had enough exposure to Ben to do an accurate assessment. Prior to our conference, Cynthia hadn't had time to check with Dr. Hartman regarding the availability of personnel to do speech therapy over the summer. But she had checked immediately afterward and had intended to contact us to convey that indeed, speech therapy for Ben could be arranged.

The last paragraph read:

Ben received appropriate services during his two semesters of enrollment in the preschool program. Most importantly for Ben, he responded posi-

*tively to them as evidenced by the gains he made. I am truly sorry that
you found your experience working with us unsatisfactory. I urge you to
continue to seek appropriate services for Ben in a facility which meets your
needs.*

There was no mention of the hearing test that wasn't done or
the treatment of the Collective Mom. Or our view of the empha-
sis on education with the dearth of attention to service. The discrepancy between Beth's informal assessment and the formal tests
was not addressed. When I read the letter, I felt no vindication or
satisfaction. I swallowed as I realized Ben could have gotten individual speech therapy over the summer. Indeed, it struck me suddenly that I'd taken a knife and slashed the rope to a lifeboat that
was tied to a powerful ship, setting my family adrift in the ocean.

Had I done Ben a service by getting him out of that environment? Or had my anger and outrage and denial taken over my
better judgment? Should I have deferred to their expertise and allowed them to measure my son's needs, trusting that they would
have helped him in the long run? Just what had I done? And
where did I go from here?

CHAPTER FIVE

Purgatory

"LET'S DANCE!" I PUSHED MYSELF OFF THE SOFA, AND BEGAN to hop and twirl around.

Ben and Peter started to giggle and shake to *A Goofy Movie*'s music in a wonderful awkwardness. I couldn't help but look down at Ben's feet, which were rigidly pointed in a toe-walking position. He'd have been a natural at ballet, but this had nothing to do with artistic expression. I caught him smiling at me and moved my arms and legs more enthusiastically. Peter's generous ears jiggled as he moved. I thought of Mr. Potato Head with two ears stuck onto each side of his face. His pacifier was held in tightly, a real feat given his big grin.

The music stopped. We fell panting onto the sofa. I hugged Peter, now almost two, next to me and stroked Ben's cheek as he sniffed his ever-present Winnie the Pooh baby blanket. It struck me how rarely Ben spoke. He interacted through gestures and one- or two-word utterances mostly. Somehow, he made his needs known to us. He frequently studied my lips when I spoke as if trying to figure out how to make the sounds and seemed to do so particularly when I spoke slowly to him. This was Ben, and these behaviors wove themselves into his other behaviors. In an odd way, it seemed normal.

I heard the door close and knew it was John coming home from his new job. He'd recently resigned his position at the mental health center. He and I talked at length about what had happened, about how he'd gone from being medical director to having employees file petty grievances against him. He was often at a loss as to how to navigate politics and when faced with conflict, John was too honest to be able to survive the entrenched powers-that-be. Still, it frustrated me. I knew how to navigate the sometimes murky political waters rather well, size people up, and articulate my thoughts. But I wasn't the one working for our livelihood.

John quickly found a new position at a local community hospital with better pay and working conditions (no travel to satellite clinics), and he'd be able to use his expertise in opening an adolescent unit for the hospital. We hoped it meant better hours as well.

John loosened his tie and suspenders, and dropped a thick envelope of hospital brochures, general employment policies, and other personnel forms on the table next to me.

"Anything important?" I said.

"Just stuff they gave me in orientation. Some of the forms that personnel has you sign for tax withholding, and other forms I know you'll file." He grinned at me before picking Peter up. Ben was hanging off his leg, smiling. So glad to see his dad home. The three of them walked into the kitchen.

I opened the envelope, separating out the papers to keep and tossing around the various glossy folders that advertised the hospital's diverse services. One pamphlet immediately caught my eye. A therapy clinic for children, with a trained pediatric speech therapist. They offered the full spectrum of services in fact, including physical and occupational therapy. The heavy feeling inside me started to lighten. The self-recriminations hadn't stopped since we'd gotten the letter from the university director a few weeks before. The days lacked structure since I'd divorced us from the preschool. I wondered each morning how much further behind Ben was. My eyes studied the brochure more slowly. My stomach started to flutter with excitement. I yelled for John.

"Did you know that the hospital had this clinic?"

He bent over and looked as I pointed at the brochure. "No."

"What do you think? I bet they could see Ben." I looked up at the clock on the mantel. After five. "I'll call tomorrow."

John nodded, reading the material.

"Did I—we—do the right thing taking Ben out of the university clinic?"

"Yes. Definitely. Ben wasn't getting what he needed." John stood to my side and snacked on an apple.

"Will he ever get caught up? I mean, you hear about these kids who don't talk until later, then they catch up, and that's it."

"He'll catch up. It'll just take more time."

"Will we ever get to the point where we have some stability?" I met his blue eyes. "It just seems so elusive. Now, a new job."

"I had no choice."

"I know." I released the words quickly. John was sensitive about the job moves. "I just wish we could be normal."

"Nobody is normal anymore. At least not the folks I'm around."

"You say that because you see depressed and psychotic people all day." I took a breath. "There are days, more and more, that I wish I could go back to work. But with your unpredictable hours and Ben's needs, it'd be impossible."

"You know how much we appreciate what you do. I know it's hard. You're very talented. Your writing is important."

"No one else thinks so." Disheartened by the continuous stream of rejections, I was thinking of giving my writing up. "Do you realize I've been getting rejected for over two years now?"

John stood up straighter. "If you want to go back to work, we'll pursue it."

"I don't think it's possible, John."

He finished his apple and sat down beside me. "It'll be okay. The hospital is a much bigger organization. There should be more buffers—more people to listen and respond to the clinicians' needs. Hopefully, more checks and balances. More accountability." He sighed, and suddenly his face looked drawn and melancholy. "Medicine is changing. Psychiatry especially. It's not like it was. Now, they have family doctors and pediatricians seeing the kids that only child psychiatrists like me used to see. And there's this backlash against physicians. Like we are just a bunch of rich, spoiled brats who've had our way too long."

"Will it get better? It's got to get better."

"I hope so."

Then he added something I almost didn't hear. "But I don't think we've seen it bottom out yet."

DAYS LATER, JOHN AND I SAT IN THE WAITING ROOM OF THE hospital children's clinic with Ben, waiting for Anju Anand, a pediatric speech therapist. I fidgeted in my seat. Thank God, John had come with me. I needed another set of eyes and ears so that later, I could bounce my perceptions off John. I didn't trust myself anymore.

The clinic was in a small gray building a couple of miles away from the main hospital. It would have been easy to drive past. The waiting room, arranged with modest chairs, had a couple of parents sitting and reading magazines. I hardly noticed. My attention was focused on Ben, and I tried to block his emotional radar from picking up my true feelings. There were large board puzzles and a few other early childhood toys in the room. After some coaxing, Ben started to play on the floor with a bucket and plastic figures.

The clock didn't seem to move. We were early, of course, but I knew some of the time would be taken up with insurance forms. I remembered when I made the appointment, the secretary had asked if it'd be all right to send for Ben's records from the university clinic. I said absolutely no, they were not to inquire or send for those documents. I had filled out some developmental history forms and sent them back so that they could be reviewed before our appointment.

Finally, I saw a woman with a light tan complexion coming toward us, smiling. I smiled back and was struck with the sincerity of her face. The woman's eyes went briefly to each of us. When she looked at Ben, it wasn't in the dissecting "what's wrong with this child?" manner that I'd come to know.

This was different.

She extended her slender hand to John and me. "Hello. I'm Anju Anand—but you may call me Anju. I'll be seeing Ben today. Why don't we go into my office and talk a bit?" Her voice was soft and lyrical, with a trace of an East Indian accent. Despite her large glasses, she was a pretty woman with wavy black hair that just touched her shoulders, and she carried a subtle confidence. Slight in frame, there was a quiet grace about her. I guessed her to be in her mid-forties.

"Hello, Benjamin," Anju said, bending slightly.

He looked away, at the floor—anywhere but her face—and remained silent. No return smile.

I helped Ben put the toys away and guided him into her office. His initial presentation always worried me. Inevitably, poor eye contact, even worse speech patterns, and inattentiveness characterized Ben when he was in a new environment. I kept murmuring that it was all right and Mommy and Daddy would stay with him the whole time.

The office was a tiny space with one medium-size desk in one corner and another, smaller desk shoved next to the opposite wall. Shelves ran up the far wall, housing games and toy sets. Ben was immediately drawn to a dollhouse in the middle of the floor and began to play while we settled into our chairs to talk. He seemed to relax, and other than checking to make sure we sat down, he separated from us easily.

"I looked over the forms you sent to us, and so perhaps we could just talk a bit more about Ben and where he is right now, the concerns you have that brought you here today." Anju cleared her throat slightly.

After a quick glance at John, I began. I told her about the delays in his speech. That was his whole problem, I emphasized. He was a bright boy. Very affectionate. I wanted to close any doors to those other diagnoses as soon as I could. I added that his initial presentation was deceiving.

John spoke to his own history of slow speech and language difficulties.

"It's his fault." I chuckled and pointed to John, then felt stupid and embarrassed.

Anju listened attentively, rarely interrupting except to clarify. She made notes during the whole time, and I caught her watching Ben as he played. She then told us she'd be testing his speech during the next few visits.

"Just speech tests, right?" I asked.

"Yes. I don't diagnose other problems. I'm only qualified to look at speech issues."

Her response earned my instant respect. I knew she was capable of addressing other problems, but she was telling me she knew her professional boundaries.

We went over some forms and one that asked for our consent to allow a student from the university clinic to observe Ben in therapy. "No," I said. "I think it would distract him too much, and he's familiar with a lot of those students."

"That is perfectly your right. You are paying for this and can choose not to have students observe." She flipped to another form in the manila folder on her desk and told us she needed a physician's referral to proceed with therapy.

John had written the initial order to evaluate. I said I would call Ben's pediatrician tomorrow and request that he write the necessary order to begin therapy.

Anju nodded, then kneeled down next to Ben and began to play with the figures in the dollhouse.

"We just got him a dollhouse for his fourth birthday a couple of months ago," I said. What I didn't add was that it had been recommended by the university preschool.

Ben watched Anju play with the dolls, sustaining attention nicely.

"Girl sleep." She put the girl doll into bed with a cover.

Ben said, "Mama go na-na." I grinned, noticing that his hair was losing some of the light blond coloring from his toddler years. But it was still curly and fine.

Anju picked up the doll. "Mama wake up."

Ben grinned, pointed at me. "Wa up."

They played for a few minutes more and then Anju stood up. "Okay. Why don't we make an appointment to start the evaluation?"

John and I agreed, and the four of us stepped into the waiting area. We said good-bye and left. It seemed too easy. I felt like I should be crying or be my usual half-hysterical self. Instead, I felt relief.

ANJU ASSESSED BEN DURING HIS FIRST TWO SESSIONS. HER experience with kids and speech difficulties was obvious. No ad nauseam Barney rhyming books here.

She explained the test results to me: Severe language disorder, both receptively and expressively. He also exhibited a moderate speech disorder that made him difficult to understand at times. Anju noted that he learned best with a combination of visual and auditory stimuli. Her plan was to see him twice a week, and she would give me instructions on how to carry over the work at home. She wanted to focus on concepts, articulation, word retrieval (helping Ben to find the words he needed to express himself), and two- to three-word sentences.

Her straightforward report, a little over two pages long, was in terms I could understand. The diagnosis: Severe Expressive Language Disorder. Anju had done two tests on Ben: the CELF-P and the Goldman-Fristoe Test of Articulation. But unlike the university clinic, she'd managed to complete both tests and determine standard scores. She didn't assess any other areas such as play skills or use the Peabody test.

For the most part, the scores were dismal. His overall composite language score (mean of 100) was 58, with his expressive score (62) slightly higher than his receptive score (50). He had multiple sound substitutions, particularly at the beginning of words (h for f, d for y, s for sh, b for l, for example). Anju concluded that his speech was intelligible 50 percent of the time. But I was amazed she could so competently assess him in such a short time. I agreed with the results, perhaps because they reflected Ben's ability to communicate and nothing more. I was ready to get started.

From then on, Ben and I went alone. Joanne watched Peter while I took Ben for his therapy. Peter suffered from frequent ear infections that seemed to get worse each time they occurred. I tried and tried to get the pacifier, which I felt literally put germs into his mouth, away from him. I had no success. It was like a blanket to him, and I wondered if he were at home more, if he'd need that extra feeling of security. The twice weekly sessions took two hours round trip, with an additional hour in therapy. By the time I picked Peter up and returned home, the kids and I were exhausted.

I sat in on the sessions with Anju and wrestled with whether I was distracting Ben. But she agreed that he needed me there for now, and she could show me how to work with him at home. I tried to keep my mouth shut and not butt in too much.

Anju sat in her chair facing me and Ben, who rested on my lap. She reached over to a large container beside her that was filled with dried beans. It looked like the kind of basin hospitals used to hold water for patients' sponge baths. I'd used quite a few of those during my nursing career, which now seemed a lifetime away.

Anju dipped a cup into the beans. "Full."

Ben's hand reached for the cup.

"Wait, Ben." She poured the beans out. "Empty. Empty."

She repeated the process. Then she let Ben play with the cup, pouring the beans back and forth.

"Enimpty."

"Good." Anju started to dip the cup into the container. Ben's hands had traveled into the beans, and he was having a great time feeling their smooth, hard shapes around his fingers and wrists. Anju pointed to her ears. "Time to listen."

Ben immediately stopped and waited. Anju filled the cup. "Full. Cup is full."

"Ull," Ben said before giggling as the hands continued to play.

Anju let him play for a few minutes, and then she moved on to some "artic" or articulation exercises. She pointed to her mouth with her index finger, rested her front teeth on her lower lip, and made the sound, "ffffffff."

Anju held up a mirror for Ben to see his mouth. His little mouth made the sound.

And so it went. Concepts such as first–last, tall–short, hot–cold, and in front of–behind were all explained and reviewed. She used a variety of toys with Ben. Small animal figures—tigers, elephants, leopards, and zebras—were positioned in various ways. The dollhouse was also used to increase sentence structure, and Anju was able to accomplish more than one objective at a time.

"Tiger in front of monkey." Her tanned slender fingers moved the tiger. "Who is behind tiger?"

Suddenly, a young boy's voice from behind the door yelled, "I can't do it, goddammit. It hurts too much."

Ben's head jerked toward the sound behind the wall. His eyes looked to me and then Anju, waiting for an explanation. "Hurt him?"

I'd seen the boy behind the voice earlier in the waiting room prior to Ben's session. He was a blond boy, around ten years old, thin, using a walker with wheels on it to enter the waiting room. His parents, both in their mid-twenties, rolled their eyes as the boy issued profanities. The room filled with his anger. I guessed him to have cerebral palsy.

I hugged Ben closer to me and tried to explain. "No. He just needs to walk to help him get stronger, and it hurts just a little bit." Ben stared at me. Another profanity came through the walls and again, Ben looked at the back of the closed white office door.

Anju spoke up. "It'll be better once we get into our new facility. We hope to move in the spring of next year. We'll have a physical therapy room. Right now, they have to walk the children up and down the hallway. I'm sorry."

I shrugged my shoulders. "It's not your fault. Ben is very sensitive to others. He's attuned to what others feel." The hallway was once again quiet, and I heard Anju redirect Ben back on task.

ANJU WORKED INTENSELY WITH BEN DURING EVERY SESSION, sharing the measurable goals with me periodically to keep me up to date. After we'd discussed them, I also signed the goal sheets, which covered the upcoming sixty to ninety days. Ben was making progress, but as with the university preschool, it was slow. The purple waters kept creeping in, especially at night.

A few days later, after dropping Peter off, I waited with Ben for Anju. I smiled at another mom who came in with her little girl. I'd noticed them before. In fact, I'd started to notice all the parents—moms mostly—and their children.

The little girl was always dressed immaculately in cute summer shorts sets. She wore braces on her lower legs and had the kind of glasses that magnified her eyes, making them appear enormous. Her brown long hair was always shiny and smooth, and pulled back in a ponytail or pigtails. Her mom sat a few seats away from Ben and me.

"Hi," I said. "Your little girl always looks so pretty."

"Thanks." She replied in a tired, but pleasant voice. She smoothed her hair—a longer version of her daughter's—away from her face. "Her name is Natalie."

I introduced Ben and told her my name.

"I'm Lynn. Natalie has spina bifida. She comes for occupational and physical therapy."

"Ben's here for speech. We come twice a week. It's about an hour's drive for us."

"Us, too." She named a town some distance away. "But at least you don't have to wait here. They get you right in. The medical center—I take Natalie at least four times a year there—makes you wait for hours. It frustrates me because you have a small child who's already anxious, and it makes for a long day. Then it's the students who see her." She sighed.

Lynn went on to tell me about the shunt in Natalie's head that helped to decrease the pressure from the excess of cerebrospinal fluid in her brain—a common problem seen in kids with spina bifida. "She's been complaining of headaches. I tried to tell them at the medical center, but they still made me wait a month for an appointment. 'Course we're on Medicaid." She shrugged her shoulders slowly as if she didn't have the energy to do it quickly. "My husband can't make too much money or we lose our health benefits for her."

"I didn't know that. That's a shame."

"Yeah. We live in a little trailer. Just the three of us."

I wasn't used to so much disclosure from someone I'd just met and yet, here in this place, it seemed appropriate. Like a world I never knew existed belonged to this place. And I realized I was a part of it. Belonged here just like every other parent and child who walked through that door. Not heaven. Not quite hell. Like a purgatory—waiting for redemption and salvation.

These parents were different from the Collective Mom. Their children were here for more than speech services. These children guided and molded the lives of their parents and their parents' future. The children's needs would be around for a lifetime. As such, we were considered patients by default.

Anju came for Ben, and I said good-bye to Lynn and Natalie.

When we arrived home a few hours later, the phone was ringing. It was my oldest sister, Leanne, who called me periodically to offer support.

We started to talk about her daughter, Katie, who was coming for a visit over her summer vacation. The boys were crazy about Katie. She was a great twelve-year-old kid. Pretty and smart, but that wasn't what made her special. What made her special was her kindness and patience. My sister and brother-in-law were invested, caring parents. We decided Katie would come for a week in July.

"Karen, you sound flat—all the time. Mom's worried about you." Leanne has a doctorate in psychology. I felt a free therapy session coming on.

"I'm okay. I just feel like crying all the time." I chuckled a little.

"You have a lot going on." She went on to listen to me vent. Then I tried to make light of it all, afraid of breaking down completely.

"You can call me anytime, you know."

"Yeah, I know. Thanks." I tried to think of something else to talk about. "How's Dad? Have you seen him this week?" Leanne lived in the same city as my parents, about two hours from Nowhere U.S.A.

"He's doing good. He's really adhering to his diet and exercise. He's so disciplined, you know?"

Yes, I did know. He'd passed that on to his daughters. From Italian immigrant parents, one of whom was illiterate, my father had instilled the love of education in his children. From the day I can remember school, I realized that learning was fundamental to one's future.

I said, "I appreciate you being so close to Mom and Dad."

"They help me, too. Now back to you, Karen. Have you thought about some antidepressant therapy? Prozac can be very effective."

"Vitamin P, eh? How's it going to help?"

"It won't take the problems away, but it might make you more able to handle them."

I took a breath. "Look, I know I'm probably depressed. But I know it's situational, okay? It's not organic." I'd worked in psych nursing and knew the lingo myself. Organic depression was when a person became depressed and couldn't figure out why. I knew why. And I knew I had all the symptoms. Overeating. Excessive fatigue. Hopelessness. Helplessness. I was a walking poster-woman for Depression.

"It doesn't have to be organic. If you're depressed, then you should do something."

"I know exactly why I'm down. It's not hard to figure it out. I just don't see a pill changing any of that." I closed my eyes and realized I'd squeezed a tear out. I hurried on, "Anyway, I appreciate your concern. Tell Ma I'm okay. Really. I'll be okay."

ANJU TAUGHT ME HOW TO DO STRUCTURED ACTIVITIES WITH Ben at home, and I tried to work with him on the days he didn't go for therapy. In addition to the speech issues and receptive issues, there were exercises for visual and short-term memory that Anju asked me to do. Occasionally, I brought home the tools that Anju had used in therapy to reinforce a concept. It seemed I was swimming as hard as I could—Ben in tow—and gaining inches, not feet. His attention span seemed to wax and wane. Some days were good. On others, he was way off task. And we still didn't know why all this was happening. Yes, he couldn't express himself, but why couldn't he understand?

I bought memory games, spent hours covering stick figure and picture diagram cards that Anju had copied from one of her books with clear Con-Tact paper and Velcro hook and eye closures. The cards were about two inches by two inches, and I attached them to a poster board to diagram sentences. On some cards, I cut out pictures of Ben, Peter, and John separately so that they could be used on the board in sentences. I chose other diagrammed pictures from Anju's book that had special meaning to Ben, like whale, shark, cat, fish, water, and swim. I stopped when I had about thirty-five cards, representing both verbs and nouns. Most were concrete concepts. But even with less specific words, the pictures gave wonderful visual cues. For example, for the verb "have," the picture showed an open hand with a big block inside it and above the picture, the word "have" was spelled out.

I called for Ben to come into the kitchen and checked on Peter, who was busy playing with his Batman figures in the living room.

"Sit here, honey," I said to Ben and positioned the white poster board upright on the table. I fixed three of the cards: a picture of Ben with his name, then a card that I'd written "loves" on, and a picture of Peter's smiling face with his name beneath. "Ben loves Peter." I pointed to each card as I said the words slowly.

Ben smiled and looked closely at the poster. "Ben la Peeda."

"Good!" I repeated the sentence, and prompted Ben to say it again.

I moved Ben to the predicate and a picture of John with "Daddy" written underneath to the subject. "Daddy loves Ben."

Ben laughed. "Daddy la Be."

"Ben." I emphasized the ending sound.

I changed the sentence to a fish as the subject, swim as the verb, and ended with the picture for water. "Fish swim in water."

Ben didn't need any prompting. "Fishie swi wata."

"Say it again, Ben."

He looked at me blankly and pointed to the cards, but seemed to have forgotten what he'd just said.

I repeated the sentence slowly.

"Fishie swim wata."

And so it went with Ben needing the constant feeding of language. He could repeat immediately after the words were said, but a delay would—most of the time—cause him to lose the utterance and become frustrated. I'd spent hours preparing the poster board and prompts, and the two of us kept at it. I found that I liked this little boy that I loved. I got to know his sense of humor, his laughter, and his easygoing nature. This would mark the beginning of many years that Ben and I would get to know each other. Our strengths and weaknesses, our most basic selves were exposed in a precious intimacy as we struggled together to make things right.

*   *   *

IT BECAME APPARENT AFTER A FEW WEEKS OF THERAPY THAT I wasn't helping Ben by sitting in on his sessions with Anju. His initial anxiety had almost disappeared. His rapport with her was excellent. He enjoyed coming. But while I was there, I was the first person he sought out if something was difficult. Anju and I decided I needed to go. A part of me was relieved. Seeing Ben struggle wasn't easy.

The day arrived when Ben would "go it alone." Anju and I had decided previously that she would come for him, and I was to stay in the chair. I was not to go back to the therapy room until it was five minutes prior to the end of the session. I'd also prepared Ben for it in the car, emphasizing that I would wait for him in the waiting room.

Anju stretched her hand out, "Come Ben, time to play."

Ben slowly stood up.

"Yes, Ben. Go with Anju. Mommy wait here whole time."

Ben took Anju's hand and started to walk down the hall. Looking ready to cry, he turned and met my eyes. I smiled and patted the chair, indicating I'd be here when he was done, and watched him finally disappear down the hallway with Anju. I swallowed and told myself he'd be fine, better off, in fact, without my presence.

Most of the magazines in the waiting room were the typical ones geared toward parents of young children. But there were others for parents of severely disabled kids. I picked one up. Pictures of kids in wheelchairs and with hand splints and Down Syndrome children at camp hit my eyes. There were ads for buying adaptive equipment. Special programs for cerebral palsy children.

Where was my son in all this? Would he be able to lead a life of independence? Get an education? Get a job? Support himself? I laid down the magazine and never picked one up again.

Every few minutes another mother with her child would file in. An infant with a naso-gastric tube in her nose. Her face didn't look quite right, but peeking out of her pink blanket was a tiny version of her mother's nose in her small face and a half-smile, fleeting, but there. A boy clinging to his mother, desperately using sign language to communicate something to her. They were such innocents and possessed a beauty because of it. I turned my eyes away, trying to block out the images that made me ache inside, and concentrated on the children's program on the TV in a corner. It didn't matter that I couldn't hear it.

As soon as it was time to check on Ben, I dashed back to the therapy room. I heard Anju's voice from behind the door, "Find monkey." A pause. "Good, Ben. Monkey under chair."

I knocked and heard a "Come in." Ben's face relaxed, "Mama!" He hugged me, and Anju was smiling.

"How'd it go?" I asked immediately after sitting down with my cuddly Ben.

"Pretty good. He was a little sad at first, and I had to redirect, but okay." Anju went on to explain what she and Ben worked on and how he'd done. "I think it will be better this way. He seemed to do well." I agreed and went home that day feeling drained.

I TOLD JOHN ABOUT BEN'S RECENT PROGRESS ON SOME OF the concepts while we were all in the car on a family diaper and dog food supply run. Everything was an hour away, but there were fewer distractions in the car. "I asked Anju if Ben might have an attention deficit problem."

"What'd she say?"

I smiled. "She was careful not to answer 'yes.' But she admitted there were times when he simply couldn't pay attention and seemed distracted. What do you think? I mean, maybe some of his memory problems are because he can't pay attention long enough to learn what he was supposed to learn. Should we try him on some Ritalin?"

John hesitated. "I'm not sure. Let me think about it. Let me spend some time with him doing different things. I'll pick things he really likes to do and some things he doesn't."

I trusted John; he'd prescribed the medicine for hundreds of children he'd assessed throughout his career. But the reason I trusted him was that he was careful not to over-prescribe, to watch the kids for side effects and, of course, to determine whether or not it was really indicated.

It was a hot summer day and the heat from the highway radiated off the pavement. The air conditioner could barely fight the humidity and high temperature. The insistent, annoying sun didn't help.

John glanced at me. "You okay?"

I realized I was gnawing on my fingernails. "Yeah. Anything new on your job? How's it going?"

"Seems to be going fine."

"Seems to be? Is it, or not?"

"It's fine."

"You always say that. You thought the mental health center was going fine, too. You think Ben's okay, as well."

"Now that's not fair," John said firmly.

We were approaching the store.

"It's not easy watching from the sidelines, just hearing what you tell me about your jobs. Then when you quit, I'm the one who stays at home, wondering what's going to happen next." I looked at John, who remained silent. I was on a roll. "Try to keep your eyes and ears open this time. Try to figure out how people are motivated. Who has the power? Who's calling the shots? Try to be a little savvier, for God's sake. And don't trust people so easily, John. Keep your boundaries up." I sighed, feeling suddenly very angry.

"I'll try. What's this really all about?" he asked.

I opened my mouth, then closed it. I'd almost told him that this job of teaching my son to speak was his fault and that if his son wasn't so much like him, maybe I could have my life back one of these days. Maybe I could get a job and not be stuck at home all day. Instead, I said, "I'm just sick of it."

John gave me one of his looks: eyebrows lifted, mouth pursed, head cocked. A cross between the psychiatrist in him and a husband who's had enough. The nonverbal equivalent of a gentle, but firm, warning that I was almost past the line of toleration.

I let what was on my mind stay there, but I couldn't help feel this increasing alienation from my husband and that he was to blame—for Ben's problems, for changing jobs, for everything. I knew that wasn't rational, but I'd grown to be obsessed about it all and where my life had taken me. As much as I loved John, I felt he and I were fighting two different battles. His was on the job. Mine was at home. And the two areas seemed to cross less and less frequently.

ONE DAY IN AUGUST, I HEARD THE DOGS' FRENZIED BARKING. They were our country doorbells. I'd have preferred a button that went "ding-dong," but it was better than nothing. The heat was unbearable, and I shot out of the house with bare feet to see if someone was coming up the drive. The boys were having an early afternoon nap.

I started down the wide cement stairs that sloped down our front yard toward the back. I stopped abruptly when I heard the hissing and saw the coiled body of a water moccasin. The sun was directly overhead, and the air was heavy and still. But I felt a chill up my arms as I realized how the boys could have come across that snake. How they often went outside without shoes on. How they could have been seriously bitten. I wasn't an expert on snakes by any means, but one of our dogs had killed a rattlesnake earlier in the year, and we'd consulted with the computer's encyclopedia— including pictures—about various snakes in the Midwest. John had mentioned that someone at work had seen a water moccasin in a regional creek, even though this type of snake was supposed to be rare in the state of Indiana. But I figured with our lake and creek, there were plenty of marshy places for snakes to nest.

Our hound, Rickie, made a grab for it, then jerked back as the snake lunged. The Labrador retriever, Nippy, kept his distance, but didn't take his eyes off the viper. Sheldon, our Shetland sheepdog, kept up an annoying high-pitched bark as a rear guard.

I remembered John telling me about his grandmother, who homesteaded a farm in the Nebraska plains. She used to carry a hoe to kill the rattlesnakes that hid in the fields.

I turned and went into the garage and picked up an old hoe in the back corner. Spitting out the spider webs that had caught in my face and blowing the dirt off the handle, I walked toward the snake, which hadn't moved from its perch on the second step. Its coiled body displayed a zigzag pattern of dull black and brown. When it opened its large mouth, I saw the white interior stretched wide. Its ugly arrow-shaped head had risen high in indignation at the howling dogs.

My stomach felt unnaturally calm as I headed toward the step. For a second the snake faced me, and I lifted the hoe high above me and swung it down with a sudden force. The concrete beneath the hoe thudded, sounding like chipped heavy glass. The snake was cut cleanly from the blade of the hoe. Its white underbelly twisted grotesquely. I continued to chop. And chop.

"Damn you." I threw the hoe down. "Damn you and everyone else for trying to hurt us. For what my son has to go through. For this emptiness inside me." When I was done and the snake lay in pieces on the step, I watched the dogs go after the remains. The sidewalk had white hack marks from my strikes, detailing each cut. I turned and walked away, thinking that no one, nothing, was going to mess with my family or me.

CHAPTER SIX

Merry Christmas

THE SUMMER WAS ALMOST OVER, AND I KNEW I NEEDED TO get my four-and-a-half-year-old Ben into another preschool soon. Kindergarten was a year away. Surely with more therapy, he'd be ready. I planned to talk to Bridget. For her own reasons, Bridget had also terminated with the university clinic. Our friendship had grown from the foundation of our sons' speech delays and membership in the Collective Mom to being able to appreciate each other as individual women, not just mothers.

I didn't know much about the local resources—I didn't have kids in the school system, I attended church sporadically, and neither my husband nor I worked in the town. Bridget was a vital source of information. She always seemed to know what was going on locally. And her two boys and mine had become great playmates. Her high energy level was daunting, and at times, I felt like a slug compared to her.

Bridget told me about a preschool just ten minutes from my house. It had such a good reputation that Bridget wasn't sure there would be any openings at this late date. I called right away and made an appointment to meet with Virginia, who ran the preschool.

A few days later, Ben and I walked inside the church, which housed the preschool, a large room in the basement of the building. I walked through the dimly lit hallway and blinked rapidly to adjust from the bright sunlight outside. Through a glossy, green-painted door, I saw a stout woman sitting at a table.

"Hi, I'm Virginia." She ran a hand quickly through her straight short hair. It landed in exactly the same place as before.

I introduced Ben and myself.

"Hello, Ben," she said with a firm, but friendly, voice.

Ben looked away. "Hi," he said in a barely audible voice. He studied the room that contained typical preschool objects—boxes of toys, a place for circle time, bulletin boards, books stuffed in bookshelves. Along one wall, cabinets surrounded a sink and counter while the opposite side of the room was brightened with large windows. Nothing seemed new or coordinated, but it was clean and as organized as the space permitted.

"Sit down," Virginia said as she stood up. "Let me get something for him to do while we talk." She returned a few seconds later with three cutout wooden puzzles, the kind with small pegs stuck into them designed for small, clumsy hands. "Here, Ben." She laid them in front of him, quickly taking the pieces out of one. I scooted his chair closer to the table.

Virginia's eyes focused on Ben for a few seconds. He put the pieces quickly back inside the first puzzle board. "Why don't you tell me a little bit about Ben."

Ben seemed unaware that he was the topic of conversation, but I kept glancing his way to make sure. I gave Virginia the usual summary of his short life. Although we hadn't had a very positive experience at the university preschool, Virginia told me other families she knew had been very pleased with their services.

"Unfortunately, we were not," I said quickly and moved on. I told her about his twice-weekly speech therapy sessions and about my hope that this preschool would help to prepare him for next fall.

"He's not autistic or handicapped," she announced after watching his progress with the puzzles. But she left unsaid her impression that there was something going on with my child. She seemed different when she interacted with Ben, warmer, softer, more gentle. Ben started to slowly explore the room, and I wondered if my own neediness made for unrealistic expectations from others.

We talked about morning sessions and luckily, there'd been a recent cancellation and thus a spot was available for Ben. School started in three weeks. The meeting lasted for a few more minutes while Virginia explained the preschool fees and that there would be an assistant for the twelve kids in the class. Twelve normal-speaking, able-to-understand kids. I inhaled and held the air inside me, exhaling slowly. Sink or swim in that normal, clear blue water the rest of the world seemed to enjoy. Could my Ben keep up? Would he even be able to float? I thanked Virginia again and left with my son.

JOHN HAD DECIDED TO PUT BEN ON A SMALL TRIAL OF Ritalin. He crushed it up and put it into a small amount of peanut butter. It was Ben's third day on the medicine. As I drove, I noticed Ben wringing his hands and staring out the window, his brows furrowed.

We came to the little bridge that crossed over our creek. "Look, Ben. Do you see any fish?" He usually enjoyed seeing the small fish swim around in the tiny pool that formed on one side of the bridge.

"I don't like that," Ben said.

My foot depressed the gas pedal, and we lurched forward. "You're doing really well with Anju. I'm proud of how you work with her without Mommy."

"I don't like that."

"I know it's hard . . ." My voice drifted off as I thought about how Ben had started his chant, "I don't like that," about two weeks ago. His fatigue was showing. At first, I saw it as a positive way for him to express himself. Then it became incessant. He said it in reaction to almost everything in his environment.

His little face turned away to look again at the gloomy fall day. The rain was quickly knocking all the leaves to the ground. No more crisp fall days to enjoy. In a few weeks, winter would bring dullness and more gray.

"I want you to work really hard with Anju today."

"I don't—"

"I want you to try!" My voice rose, and my hands fisted around the steering wheel. "Quit saying, 'I don't like that'! Don't you like anything?"

He met my eyes before twisting his fingers some more. The rain became stronger so I turned the headlights on. Inside the car, I batted my eyes to keep the tears from obscuring my vision and thought how very little I liked my own life.

ABOUT FORTY-FIVE MINUTES LATER, I GREETED THE CLINIC'S staff. "Good morning." I signed Ben's name on the clipboard as "Patient In" and checked the ST box for speech therapy.

"Hey there." A smiling chubby woman with brown hair and glasses looked up from behind the counter. "How's Ben today?"

"He's okay. The rain's really bringing down all the pretty leaves." Our area of the state was widely known for its fall foliage. Millions of people came yearly to shop and unwind in the small quaint town.

"My husband and I need to go out your way before they all fall off," she chuckled.

She was the clinic's receptionist and coordinated all the billing and generally kept the place organized. Fortunately, John's new insurance was authorizing and paying for the majority of the speech sessions. Another familiar face smiled at me as she folded towels. This lady's job as technician to the therapists was a cornucopia of miscellaneous, yet important duties, ranging from making sure the supplies were replenished, fresh towels were available, and all the equipment was put away. Each time I came, these women welcomed me, and treated me with respect and kindness, and Ben with warmth and caring. Slowly, I'd gotten to know them, and a little about their children and family life.

It was comforting to see their faces when I came. Somehow, it helped me to feel like more than just a part of some Collective Mom. I read again the framed saying on the wall. It had to do with how the clinic appreciated the child first and recognized the handicap second. Ben and I sat down, and I placed my hand in his little warm one. "It'll be all right," I whispered.

He met my eyes and didn't say, "I don't like that."

AFTER WATCHING BEN FOR A FEW MORE DAYS, IT WAS OBVI-ous the Ritalin had no positive effect on our son. It only increased his general anxiety that seemed to have escalated with the intro-duction of preschool. So we stopped giving it to him. His hand-wringing stopped as well. A part of me was relieved, while another had hoped—perhaps—the answer could be found in a pill.

The first day of preschool represented Ben's first, ongoing con-tact with other kids his age who had no delays. It seemed a bit easier than the university clinic. Perhaps he sensed no one was evaluating or watching him. Or perhaps it was because he was a year older. The first weeks proceeded without major incident. There was the usual repeated questioning by Ben, "You come back?" Other than that, he seemed to enjoy going.

But after Ben had been going to the school for about two months, I became aware of an increase in his anxiety. It was as if the social aspects of the school were overwhelming him. I tried to put myself in his place, unable to speak and understand with the same skills as his peers. Every morning, I reassured him, talked about what he liked about school, and distracted him by remind-ing him of coming home later in the day.

On Mondays, Wednesdays and Fridays, the days Ben had his two and a half hours of morning preschool, I took Peter with me to pick Ben up. This was a particularly blustery fall day, the kind that happens when the leaves are brittle underfoot, and the first one that creates the need for jackets and lightweight coats. I watched the leaves blow in small masses and the trees bend angrily at having to shed their splendid colors. I pulled our van into the gravel lot. There was Ben, on the playground next to the church.

But he'd seen me first, as usual. His tiny fingers wrapped around the chain link fence, his head turned, waiting for sight of our car and me to come for him. And as usual, he was alone. The other kids swung on the swings, played tag, crossed the wooden bridge, and fought imaginary wars. Mine stayed by the fence, waiting for me.

I stepped out of the car with Peter in my arms, who was begging to play. "No, Pete, we have to get home." I didn't think my two-year-old could hold his own; some of the kids played pretty roughly.

There were four other moms waiting around, chatting. I felt different. I was older than most of them. Some were "locals," having known one another their entire lives. All their kids could talk and understand what was said to them.

Virginia took her post by the gate that allowed her to see each child safely off with his parent or grandparent. She seemed to use the station as a communication vehicle for parents. A couple of weeks ago, she'd gently chastised me for not orienting Ben to the fine art of board games and turn-taking. As far as I was concerned, I was lucky that he'd finally mastered the concepts of first—last with Anju.

Today, as soon as I was within speaking distance, Virginia leaned on the fence and said, "Ben couldn't find his coat this morning. And I didn't know which one was his. He had no idea which one it was. So I let him put that one on." She pointed to my son who'd arrived at the gate. "I think it's a girl's coat, though."

The other moms stopped talking and turned to me.

I swallowed and felt a rush of heat in my cheeks. "I just got a new one out of the closet for him. I probably should have made sure he knew what it looked like." I thought of the dimly lit hallway outside the preschool room, a wall lined with hooks and crowded coats with barely enough light to differentiate dark colors. But I assumed Ben would be able to recognize his little green jacket. I should have labeled it. I should have pointed it out to him. Made sure he knew which one was his. The echo of Shitty Mother sounded.

Ben moved toward the half-opened gate, smiling.

"Hi, Benny. Where'd you get that coat?" It was a denim coat with a rhinestone heart to one side. Obviously, it was a girl's jacket.

He looked at it. "Don't know."

"Well, take it off, and let's go in and find yours." I slipped him through the gate and took him inside. "Take off that one, Ben." He quickly took it off. "Here's yours, honey. Don't you remember, it's green with a zipper?"

After stepping outside again with Peter still pulling at me to get down, I thanked Virginia, made my face freeze into a smile as I nodded to each of the other moms, who turned as I exited, and got the kids situated in the van. I turned the corner, looked back to make sure no one could see me and started to cry.

SOMEHOW I'D MANAGED TO SNEAK AWAY TO CHICAGO FOR A couple of days to stand up at my friend's wedding. Rosa and I had met six years earlier, during my single, Ph.D. days at the University of Illinois. Our friendship since that time had solidified through phone calls or yearly visits, and she'd listened more times than I wanted to count about my struggles with Ben.

I'd flown to Chicago on a short flight from Indy, and Rosa had excitedly met me at the airport. We drove to the condo she and her fiancé, Jeff, shared on the near-north side of the city. No burbs for this girl. We'd settled in after dinner, and Jeff had gone to bed. Girl time. I sat across from Rosa, crossed-legged on the couch, with a story I wanted to enter in a new magazine, *The Family Circle/Mary Higgins Clark Mystery Magazine*.

Rosa sipped her tea—what I called her tree tea. It had these sticklike things in it. She assured me it was natural and much healthier than anything I'd given my body in years. She was probably right. Although Pop-Tarts were supposed to have vitamins.

"I don't get the beginning. Why wouldn't the doctor just call the unit?" Her almost black eyes gazed at me, and then her fingers quickly flipped to another part of the story. She was of Puerto Rican descent and bilingual, able to switch back and forth, much like her persona. A girl one minute, bouncing her black corkscrew hair up and down, and then, a mature, worldly woman the next, ready to go to work in a jacket and skirt at her government office where she handled millions of dollars.

I made a note in the margin. "I see. Okay. What else?"

She gave frank, unyielding, often brutal feedback—the kind every writer craves after so many rejections offering nondescript messages such as "not right for us," "just didn't fall in love with it," or simply, "I'm passing on this one." Last summer, I'd gone to a university writers' conference, feeling much like a fool with my mystery and thriller pieces when most of the other workshop participants had come with literary works in hand. But the workshop leader had been kind and reassuring. It was then that I knew I didn't really know much about writing. Concepts such as pacing, dialogue, finding the "center to a story," and areas of tension were new vocabulary words that I began to understand. And I kept writing.

Rosa told me the protagonist wasted too much time in the beginning of the story, a minor character wasn't necessary, and the middle was confusing. I thanked her profusely.

She laid the papers down. "How's Ben doing?"

I inhaled. "I think he's making progress. Anju is so great. She works her butt off with him. Preschool is so-so. The teacher's assistant has been kinda looking out for him. He's just so damn scared to be there. At home, he's like another kid. Relaxed. Funny. When I try to tell people this, they're like 'right, uh huh. Another mom in denial.'"

"That little boy is so perceptive. He knows. You can tell he knows."

"That's what John says. He says all you have to do is look in the eyes and you can tell he's clicking." I looked away. "I think I'll call John again."

"Kare, you just called him last night."

I stopped looking in my purse for my calling card.

Rosa shrugged her shoulders. "Okay, girl. I'm not talkin' you out of it."

John told me he'd broken a crown off a back tooth, Ben was sick and had thrown up all night, and it looked like Peter was getting sick. I hung up feeling guilty and torn. Glad to be in Chicago and wishing I was home. Rosa quickly whisked me off for a day in the city. We rode the El, shopped at Marshall Field's and Neiman-Marcus. Jeff took us for a drive at night, a beautiful clear night where the Navy Pier was lit up like a giant gangplank extended from a magical pirate ship.

The next day, the wedding went beautifully. It was pure Rosa and Jeff. A unique, classy affair that was what they wanted it to be. Their life together was theirs to make. I felt honored to have been a part of it, but wondered if I was saying good-bye to a part of our friendship.

When I arrived at home, I got back to work with Ben. I sent the revised story to the magazine, beating the deadline by a week.

ALTHOUGH BEN HAD ALWAYS LOVED WALKING AND RUNNING, HE was a bit clumsy. One October night, he'd taken a tumble on the stairs, breaking his collarbone. We had given the boys their baths and put them to bed for the night. About half an hour later, we were startled to hear a little boy's sobs from the stairwell. After discovering Ben at the bottom of the stairs, holding his arm and crying, he told us, "I thirsty."

The emergency room physician had been pleased with how co-operative Ben had been with the X ray and examination. John had stayed with Ben, and I'd helped keep a sleepy Peter occupied in the waiting room. The doctor informed us that a padded strap that wound around Ben's shoulders would be all that was needed to ensure proper healing of the bone. Sure enough, the follow-up X ray a few weeks later confirmed this.

Also in November, Anju told me she needed to take some time off. Would I consider another therapist to avoid the three-week interruption in therapy?

"No. Ben's really bonded to you. He's making good progress, and to be honest, he needs a break as well." The "I don't likes" had stopped, but he was tired. Preschool, and the anxiety it caused, drained him. He came home, ate hungrily, and napped for two hours.

"That's fine." Anju cleared her throat. "There's a goal review due, and I thought we'd go over Ben's treatment plan together. I'll send it to Ben's physician for his signature. Your insurance has approved twelve more sessions."

I sat next to her and studied the sheet in front of me. Ben's diagnosis was listed as "Speech/Language Disorder." Color and shape identification; sequencing action pictures; and labeling categories such as body parts, modes of transportation, and furniture were on the plan for the upcoming three months. Both understanding the concepts and expressing them were interwoven into the goals.

I read Anju's summary of my son's treatment thus far:

Ben has achieved all goals from previous treatment plan. His processing, as well as his verbal skills, is improving very well. Attention has significantly improved needing no redirection throughout the session. He has received 37 sessions to date. Continue with ST 1–2 x a week.

"Sounds good. He's talking a lot more at home."

Anju nodded. "Yes, he's making excellent gains."

"You know," I said softly, "I was talking to his preschool teacher, and he's not where he should be as far as holding a pencil—it's difficult for him to trace his name and cut with scissors. What do you think about some occupational therapy? Could we coordinate the therapy sessions so that it'd be on the same days?"

"I think so. I can talk with Elizabeth, our OT, and see what her schedule is like."

I thanked Anju again, wondering if she knew just how grateful I was, and stood up. "I'll see you in December, then." Ben and I got into the car and headed for Burger King. The car could have found the place without my steering. It was a small treat after his hard work, and he loved fast food.

In the drive-through, I waited for the voice behind the speaker box to acknowledge me. Ben seemed fairly content today, and I squeezed his hand and smiled. While I acknowledged his progress, it seemed so slow. A drop in the vast bucket of his language delay. I saw him during those preschool days, unable to keep up, clutching the fence in anticipation of my coming for him. My uneasiness was also increasing due to concerns over his safety and emotional well-being. Did he belong with "normal" children? Should I place him with others who were delayed? John had said no, that it would only increase his problems. Then there was the testing that would have to be done to place him with other kids who were delayed. All I knew was that my son was four and a half and lucky to get a noun, verb, and object into one sentence.

A garbled voice interrupted my thoughts, and I placed my food order.

THE BREAK OVER THANKSGIVING FLEW BY. AS ALWAYS SEEMED to happen, the holiday rush made my to-do list longer than Santa's. Then Virginia announced a children's program the week before Christmas and gave instructions for appropriate attire. A few days later, we wrapped the kids up in coats and mittens, and set out in the dark night to see the program and hear the carols.

As soon as I entered the large, lower-level room where the kids would be singing, I saw Virginia herding the kids behind the stage. I gave Ben a hug and released him to Virginia's direction. The metal folding chairs were filling up quickly, and we settled Peter, now almost two and a half, next to John with instructions to "be quiet."

Peter's verbal skills had exploded and if formally assessed, he probably would have scored higher than Ben on language tests.

But even suspecting this discrepancy, I didn't compare the boys too much. To me, they were just Ben and Pete, with a right to be what they were.

I put my finger to my lips, "Shhh," and made steady eye contact with Peter for a few seconds. His clear blue eyes looked back at me, trying to size up how serious I was. The tense look on my face must have convinced him because he started to innocently study the crowd.

The basement air was stuffy and stifling. But that wasn't what made my lungs feel tight. I knew Ben was anxious, really anxious. He'd been unusually quiet and still, looking out the van window during the drive. I had this sense of foreboding. Something felt off. I had to consciously shake the intense desire to stand up, grab the kids, and run home.

But the noise from the room pushed me down into my seat. I stretched to see if I could glimpse Ben behind the curtain. There were just a few shadows of small bodies being lined up. Finally the show started. The youngest kids sang their songs first. It sounded like a mix of monks chanting and being yelled at by fifteen four-year-olds. Mercifully, it ended fairly quickly.

Ben's class was next. I saw him near the back—due to his height—kind of stuck into the corner. Something seemed to lift me from the chair, and I kept my eyes focused on him as I went to stand by the stage. I waved at him. He saw me, his body rigid. He nodded and gave me a quick wave as if he couldn't spare any attention from the tasks at hand. I wanted to cry and felt like a complete fool. I turned around. The crowd's voices blurred and grew louder. Smiling faces melted into one big mass. Then silence.

The first song commenced. Ben mouthed a few words, but stopped and started throughout the song. A second song began. In addition to carrying the tune, the kids were supposed to step around the stage. A circle was formed with each child stepping from carpet square to carpet square. Ben's turn came, and he stopped. The whole group bumped up against him. He didn't know what to do. Another boy whispered something to him. A girl nudged the line.

Out of the corner of my eye, I saw Virginia's assistant come onto the stage and guide my son from carpet to carpet. She took his hand and pointed what to do. Ben responded to her visual cues, a bit awkwardly and timidly, but the kids were able to continue. The rest of the recital passed in a blur. I'd set my son up for failure. Because of my pride, I'd expected too much. I shouldn't have expected him to keep up. As soon as Ben left the stage, I went back to my seat.

After the boys drank a quick glass of syrupy punch and ate a couple of dry cookies, we left. The night had gotten colder and darker. I begged John to hurry and unlock the doors for the kids and me. We threw ourselves in and buckled our seat belts. Between chattering teeth, I told Ben, "Mama is so proud of you tonight. You did great."

His eyes assessed me. "Tanks," his voice was soft and I couldn't help but think he didn't believe me.

Through the night, I hadn't paid much attention to John. He sat stiffly behind the steering wheel, and I asked, "What did you think?"

"He did all right."

"He didn't know what the hell he was doing." My voice was low.

"I know." A pause. "I know." His voice cracked.

My head whipped around to look at the profile of my husband. Although John's denial had been irritating and contradictory, it had fueled the faith inside me. He was a child psychiatrist. If he thought his son would be okay, I could still hope so, too.

But John's answer tonight was different. He couldn't deny anymore. The loss was bitter, and I felt a shared grief with this man whom I loved and a terror at what we were facing.

"What are we going to do?" I asked.

"I have faith in him. We do what we've been doing. That's all we can do."

"Are you sure?"

Silence.

I wiped my face, now wet, and heard a tiny voice from behind me. "Daddy, why is Mommy sad?" It was Peter.

I interrupted before John could reply. "I'm not sad, honey. I think Ben did a terrific job. I'm so proud—of both of you." I swallowed, desperate for my voice to carry a conviction that I didn't feel. "You listened really well tonight, Pete."

Ben's small voice said, "I okay?"

I cleared my nose. There was no way I was going to let those kids or John see me cry any more tonight. I turned my full face toward Ben. "You did really well. And you know what, Ben? I love you and Peter and your daddy very much."

He exhaled and the air around his mouth was momentarily surrounded by a white cloud.

"Okay, honey?" I asked, reaching to squeeze his mitten.

"I sang some songs."

"Yes, you did, Ben. And they were beautiful."

JUST BEFORE CHRISTMAS, AND AFTER MY REQUEST FOR A RE-ferral, our pediatrician ordered an occupational therapy evaluation. He agreed with me and thought it was a good idea, since kindergarten would begin in six short months. So at four years and eight months, Ben's fine motor skills were formally assessed. The conclusions: "Generalized upper extremity weakness; and difficulty with drawing/writing tasks, and some fine motor and self-care activities." His writing was very light, his fingers unable to press down on the page. He preferred finger foods.

I had mixed feelings about the addition of more therapy. I knew Ben needed it. He'd never liked to color or draw. And I wasn't surprised that these skills were weak. I didn't know if his broken right collarbone of a few months earlier—Ben's dominant hand was right—had exacerbated his delays or not. I also felt that I had some time before kindergarten started. I felt ahead of the game in a way.

In another sense, I felt increasingly overwhelmed with adding yet another therapy and another area to keep track of. His delays seemed to grow more complex and multifaceted. Since the Christmas pageant, my anger had subsided. I felt that I'd better get with the program, so to speak, for my son's sake and for the family's sake. I decided that I was fortunate to have this clinic for my son, and our insurance carrier was authorizing payment for both therapies.

The OT goals were straightforward: increasing grip strength; successfully using a tripod grasp on his pencil (a small three-sided plastic device that slid onto the pencil and allowed him to grasp it more easily); increasing movement from wrist to hand; copying a plus sign; putting on his own socks; exerting more pressure when he wrote; and continued assessment of visual perceptual and visual motor skills. Ben would be seen in OT once a week.

I liked Elizabeth, Ben's occupational therapist, as much as I liked Anju. She was about my age and had two young sons in grade school. I didn't feel bad when I told her what Ben wasn't able to do. Her brown hair touched just below her ears, and she had a pretty open face with sensitive and responsive green eyes.

She gave me ideas on how to work with Ben at home. Alligator scissors, the kind you squeeze to make the blades come together, would help to increase his hand strength. She gave me some "therapy-putty," a red stretchy, rather firm substance that he could shape and mold. Small objects, like a penny, could be hidden inside for him to dig through and find. Elizabeth suggested we get him a clipboard to help stabilize the paper, guide his fingers in tactile name and letter tracing, have him do mazes, roll a rolling pin, and use Colorforms—those movable plastic cutouts with a background scene.

The new routine was for Anju to see Ben first, and then walk him to Elizabeth's room for an hour of OT. Given that I had two hours while Ben was in therapy, I began to run errands on those days. It gave me time to breathe, if only for a short time. And I was proud of Ben, who'd been able to walk with Anju down the hall to Elizabeth's office without getting anxious about my absence in the waiting room. Elizabeth reported he was tired after Anju, but willing to work.

One day, I arrived back at the therapy clinic and waited for Ben to finish with Elizabeth. The clinic had finally moved into their new building. It was ten minutes farther away for me to drive, but to say the new facility was an improvement would have been an understatement. The physical therapy area was enormous. OT and ST offices and rooms had been added. A bigger, brighter waiting room for the kids made the children more at ease. And although the walls and carpet still smelled of new construction, the staff had made a wonderful collage of the children's hand-prints on the hallway wall. All the little hands were stamped with bright red, blue, green, pink, purple, and orange paint. Ben's was there, one of the largest of the red handprints.

Ben smiled at me through the glass of the new waiting room. Elizabeth grinned, too, and sat down beside me to give me a re-port of what they'd worked on that morning. "He is such a dear. I want you to know your son has a wonderful sense of humor." She glanced at Ben, fondness evident in her eyes. "We did something different this morning. I wrapped Ben up in a mat on the floor, and he pretended he was a hot dog. I compressed my hands on his joints. As I pushed down, I told him I was putting ketchup, mus-tard, and pickle relish on him."

I must have looked puzzled.

"This is helpful for body awareness and proprioceptive input prior to motor planning activities." She gestured with her hands and paused briefly. "It means Ben needs to have more awareness of his body's movement in space as he interacts with his environ-ment. I think Ben has some SI issues, sensory integration. It's where the child lacks this body awareness, among other things. A child with SI has trouble integrating all the stimuli from his en-vironment efficiently."

"I see." I looked at Ben, his legs swinging up and down under his chair. "Get chicken and French fries?" The question was a rare and well-articulated five-word utterance for Ben.

"Yes, Ben, but let me talk to Elizabeth now."

She continued to explain SI, and it made some sense, I supposed.

During the ride home, I thought about what Elizabeth had said in relation to behaviors I'd seen from Ben. Although Ben ate a lot—he was still very big for his age—he was very particular about what he ate, as if unable to tolerate different textures of food. He had a sensitive gag reflex, but I wasn't sure if that was related to SI in any way. Pizza was his all-time favorite food with fast food being a close second. He also carried his Winnie the Pooh blanket around everywhere when he was at home. Having it beside him constantly, I'd watch him stroke and smell it intermittently, as if squeezing sensory stimulation from it. Athletically, Ben was awkward, unable to jump rope or catch a ball very well. His legs, however, had firm muscles from hours of walking and running around our backyard. He was also clumsy, as evidenced by many spills and falls during his short life.

Last, he was acutely sensitive to loud sounds. We'd stopped being able to go to the theater as a family. John would usually take Peter to see a movie while I stayed with Ben. Ben's hearing sensitivity seemed to cause him physical pain. Once, we'd gone shopping and entered an electronics store. The stereos blared from the back with deep bass reverberations. Ben quickly cupped his hands over his ears and begged us to leave. From then on, he refused to go into stores that played loud music.

THE LIGHTS CAME ON AT ABOUT FIVE-THIRTY A.M. CHRISTMAS morning. Peter woke Ben up, and I saw them standing side by side at the top of the stairs. Peter wore his red Robin pajamas (as in Batman) and Ben wore a pair of soft blue plaid ones. John was ready, video camera in hand, taping this moment when magic is totally believed in. Ben slid out of sight for a minute.

"Pete, where's Ben?" I asked.

"He's here. He's right here." Peter's voice had a higher pitch to it and was funny just to listen to.

"Well, come on, guys." They followed me closely down to the kitchen. I stopped abruptly and felt one of them knock into me. "Look! The cookies are gone. Santa must have eaten them." I looked at the two boys' faces, frozen in awe. John coughed and grinned, as if reminding me of the stale cookies he'd tasted the night before.

"Wait." I touched their arms gently. "Do you think he left anything for you guys?"

Peter ran into the dark living room. I hurried to turn on the lights, but dimmed them to allow the Christmas tree's lights to add color and warmth to the room. I knelt down and started to hand out packages. Each boy went to his respective position to stack his stash. Peter took the loveseat and ripped with a fury. "Baman!" It was a plush Batman figure, complete with cape and mask. "I love Baman."

Then on to a Huff'n Puff vacuum cleaner. "Vacuum," Peter yelled, being my neat and orderly boy who loved to clean. I hoped some woman would one day appreciate my cultivating such domestic talent.

"Santa told me it really works if you put batteries in it," I told Peter in a confidential tone. My direct contact with Santa humbled him for a millisecond before he tore into another present.

Ben was also pleased with Santa's purchase decisions. "Oh boy, tanks, Dad. A spaceshippie. Open? Open?" He eagerly bent over it, examining the box carefully.

"After all the presents are opened, honey," I said.

Peter got some Play-Doh and a book. Crayons and paper. Ben got a new Toy Story Colorform set and started to open another box.

"What'd you get, Ben?"

"Car. Car. Open?"

"Just wait. After all the presents are unwrapped." I picked up one of the last ones under the tree for the kids. "Here, Ben."

"I no wanna more." He was happy with his pile of presents and was busy looking inside the Star Wars packages. "Open?"

"Pretty soon." I kissed him on the cheek. "One more for you, Ben."

"Tanks." He reached for it and opened a child's suitcase, the kind with a long handle and two wheels for easy pulling. Back to his spaceships.

"Here, Pete." I handed him his suitcase—and realized I'd become my mother, buying identical or near identical items for my kids.

Peter tore the red Christmas wrap aside and felt the vinyl on the outside of the case. "A tablecloth! Thanks."

John, still waking up, peered from behind the camera. "What'd he say?"

"He thinks it's a tablecloth because of the vinyl," I said, laughing, and went over to Peter, who'd just torn off the last piece of paper. "No, it's a suitcase. For when we go on vacation."

Peter looked at me, the suitcase, then back at me. "Oh, okay." He shoved it aside and admired his vacuum cleaner once again. "Where are the batteries?"

SPEECH THERAPY CONTINUED AFTER THE HOLIDAYS. BEN AND I were waiting for Anju to come for us one day. I saw her in the hallway and put my magazine down. As she came closer I noticed immediately that she was wearing a wig. Ben looked curiously at it.

"You can touch it," she said kindly. "It's a wig. A wig."

Ben reached up to touch it gently. He reached again and smiled. "Wig."

All the missed appointments made sense now, and I was overwhelmed with sadness for her. And so much admiration. She had hidden her illness from us, never letting on that she was worried about anything or didn't feel well.

"I didn't know you were ill."

We talked a little about it, and I waved good-bye to Ben as he left with Anju.

Had there been no signs of illness, or had I become so wrapped up in my own life that a perverse selfishness existed inside me? I felt out of touch with my nieces and nephews, sometimes with my parents. There just didn't seem to be anything left over. Rosa had been patient, but I wondered if our lives were diverging too quickly and too widely. Downtown Chicago versus seventeen acres in the country. A high-powered, full-time job versus a stay-at-home mom. I lived in the world of purple water and it seemed that world owned me—at least for now.

I crossed my legs, finding it difficult to sort out the feelings of guilt and sadness. Then, Natalie, the little girl with spina bifida, wheeled herself into the waiting room using a motorized wheelchair. Her mother, Lynn, and a physical therapist walked in beside her. The efficient whir of the chair's motor was interrupted only by the clicks of the start and stop command.

My breathing became forced. Nothing made any sense. The little girl's loss of mobility was unfair. Why wasn't she walking anymore? Hadn't the physical therapy helped? Had something happened?

Lynn came up to me, grinning. I'd never seen her face come close to a smile before.

"Isn't it great? Medicaid finally approved the chair. Now she can leave the house. She can go to the mall and see everything. We used to go, and she'd get so tired, we'd have to leave. Now she can go anywhere." Her long dark hair fell across her shoulders as she bent down toward her daughter. We all started to watch the physical therapist check and tighten attachments to the chair.

I closed my mouth. The realization of what the chair meant to Natalie in terms of socialization and extended mobility began to sink in. I had to admit it was a wonderful chair with deep blue padding, built just for this girl's little body. Natalie, with her glasses that made her eyes appear enormous and pigtails that jiggled when she nodded, maneuvered the controls like a racecar driver.

"She just loves it," Lynn said.

"That's great," I murmured, watching Natalie tell the physical therapist when the adjustment made her legs more comfortable.

I shook my head and stood up to leave. Anju's illness. Natalie's wheelchair.

I left wondering if anything was as it seemed.

CHAPTER SEVEN

Inertia

"OKAY, GUYS, PLEASE BE QUIET. MAMA'S GOT TO ANSWER THE phone." I hurried over at the third ring, hoping it was John. I glanced at my watch: four o'clock.

"Hello." I ignored Peter's whine in the background.

"May I speak with Karen Foli, please?" It was a woman's voice. I guessed it was a solicitor.

"Who is this?" My voice was not friendly.

"This is Kathy Sagan, editor-in-chief of *The Family Circle/Mary Higgins Clark Mystery Magazine.*"

My hands started to perspire and feel slippery against the receiver. "This is Karen Foli."

"I'm calling to let you know your short story, 'A Danger to Others,' won first place in the Mary Higgins Clark Mystery/ Suspense Short Story Contest. We just loved it. Mary made the final decision, but it was unanimous by the committee. It's a wonderful story."

It took a while for my brain to register that "Mary" was Mary Higgins Clark. My God, Mary Higgins Clark had read my story, my words. "Are you kidding?"

"No." Kathy Sagan chuckled. "Mary especially liked the scene with the little boy and the doctor. It was very touching."

"Thank you." I exhaled. "You're not kidding. Thank you so much."

"You're welcome. We'll need some biographical information to put with the story and a picture of you. Do you have a picture?"

"I'll get one. This is just wonderful. You have no idea what this means to me." I covered the mouthpiece with my hand. "Peter, stop it!" I put my mouth back up to the phone. "Can you hold for just a second?"

"Peter, please, be quiet. I'll be done in a minute. Just a few minutes." I gently shooed him away, putting my fingers to my lips. He started to cry, but I turned my back to him. "Sorry about that. My little boy isn't cooperating." I could hear the embarrassment in my apology. "I'm just a little curious. How many entries did you have?"

The soft voice with a faint New York accent continued. "There were fifteen hundred stories entered. We hope for a circulation of around half a million, but we'll see. Your story will appear in the spring issue." She paused. "Do you have any other questions?"

"Not right at the moment. Can I get your number?"

Peter yelled for something on the kitchen counter he couldn't reach. I would have given him my fine china to quiet him if it had been close by.

She read off her phone number, her assistant's number, and the amount of the prize money. I hung up, dazed, thinking back to the fall visit in Chicago and Rosa's help with the story. I recalled putting it in the mail, believing the odds of winning were so slim that I was wasting the envelope and stamp. And I particularly remembered all those days when I was ready to quit writing. Although I had written two books and had a good start on a short-story collection, the rejection letters continued to pile up.

I wiped my hand over my forehead and stopped. It dawned on me that I'd bought the magazine and found out about the contest because of Ben's speech therapy. We'd stopped at a bookstore on the way home as a treat. Maybe things happened for a reason.

Then I looked at Peter, who, the minute I'd hung up the phone, had found a toy to play with. I grabbed his little hands and started to jump around the kitchen. I jumped and jumped, and laughed and shouted. Peter broke away, and he and Ben gave each other looks that said, "Mama's gone crazy." But with each shout and jump, that shrunken inner kernel of what used to be Karen grew stronger, and told me that she was still alive.

BY THE END OF MARCH, MY STRESS WAS INCREASING IN AN-ticipation of the coming year of kindergarten. Ben was leaving the world of developmental delays and entering a world of academics. He wasn't ready, and I knew it.

One Sunday afternoon, John and I had arranged for a sitter to watch the boys while he and I ran errands in a nearby town. Rather than go to the usual city, we headed in the opposite direction. The early spring day appeared dull and still, all life hiding or sleeping until warmth came. A few miles from home, I noticed a couple of white buildings with a playground in back of one of the structures.

"What are those buildings?" I pointed.

"I'm not sure. I think it's a school."

Before whizzing past, I read the sign. It was a Montessori school. "I didn't know this was here." I looked at the time. "It's only about twenty-five minutes from the house. I wonder if they have a kindergarten."

"You can always call and ask."

"He'd be safer there, don't you think? I mean, maybe they wouldn't put him through all those tests again, like the public school would." I turned around in my seat, as the school grew smaller in the distance. "Ben said a little boy kicked him in the stomach at preschool the other day. Remember, I told you?"

John turned sharply. "Yeah, I remember."

My mouth grew dry. Ben couldn't tell me what had happened. He was able to tell me who had kicked him and that he'd been kicked, but nothing else, really. He couldn't tell me if he'd been fighting or just playfully wrestling. He had been very upset, though, and I could tell it hurt a lot.

I started to bite my fingernail, but stopped myself. "I called Virginia, and she said that she hadn't known about it, but the boy had been aggressive with other children."

"She didn't think it was Ben's fault, did she?"

"No. She immediately told me there'd been another parent who'd complained about that boy."

"Where was Virginia when Ben got kicked?" John's voice had gone from the relaxed tones of a man on a drive to the firmness of a doctor considering a patient.

"She was out there watching the kids, but it's a pretty big area, and there are places that aren't easily seen." I sighed. "It was scary because I knew someone had hurt Ben, but I couldn't tell Virginia any more than that."

John's lips were set in a hard line. Since the Christmas pageant, he'd been even more protective of Ben. I'd watch him give Ben an extra hug and kiss at night, and when John would pull away, I'd see sadness in my husband that hadn't been there before.

I crossed my arms. "I want him to be safe. That's all I want right now. He's been through so much."

"Give this school a call. Get some information. Whatever he needs, that's what we'll do," John said.

I CALLED THE SCHOOL THE FOLLOWING WEEK AND FOUND OUT that there were several preschool programs, a kindergarten and an elementary school. I made an appointment to tour the school. When the day arrived, I dropped the kids off at Joanne's house and drove up the highway to the school.

I walked up to the designated building, opened a door marked "Administrative Office," and was greeted by a middle-aged woman with a bright smile. Her very short hair framed her cheerful face, and she greeted me with an outstretched hand. "Hello, I'm Nancy Madison. You must be—should I call you Mrs. Thompson or Ms. Foli?"

"Either one is all right." I'd given up some of my defensiveness from the university clinic days, but I thought it was nice of her to ask. My desperation to help Ben had humbled me considerably.

Nancy had the air of someone who felt so comfortable in her job that it was like a second home. She was one of those lucky people who were able to stay in a job for decades because they chose to.

"Why don't we do the tour first? Then you can ask questions as you think of them."

"Great."

She walked around her desk, and I inventoried the small office: a light green metal desk, filing cabinets, and a closet-like room behind it with a copy machine. Nothing fancy. It looked exactly like what it was—a small private school's front office. We left this suite and went down a short hallway.

"This is our pre-preschool program. It's for small children around eighteen months to about three years."

There was an archway into the room with a short white fence in front of it. My hand moved to the arch, and I peered into the room, my eyes resting on a group of small children eating fruit bars around a table. Two children with straight, coal-black hair— of Asian descent—and a child with tanned skin and silky black hair, briefly glanced my way. A little girl with curly hair and skin the color of coffee with cream sat daintily on the floor, and a Cau- casian child joined her to play.

It was a mini United Nations. Twenty-two minutes from my home in the middle of Nowhere U.S.A. was a wonderfully diversified classroom, full of small children from many ethnic backgrounds. Besides being absolutely beautiful, the children were darn cute as well. Like all the children I'd see that day, it was obvious their mothers and fathers had carefully dressed them, combed and braided their hair, and kissed them good- bye.

"I had no idea this was such a culturally diverse school." I couldn't take my eyes off the room, sprinkled with bold bright colors and low shelves perfect for short bodies. "But it's wonderful," I added quickly.

"Due to the Fortune 500 companies in this city, employees are recruited from around the world—Japan, India, Australia, Germany. Many of their children come here to school." Nancy stopped to answer a staff member's question.

I watched while a small girl, with beautiful eyes and a tuft of hair sticking upright from a red bow, removed a tray from one of the shelves near the arch. She stopped and studied me. I grinned, and she shyly grinned back, grabbed the tray, and hurried toward the center of the room. I wanted to take her home.

Nancy and I proceeded to the next room, one of three preschool areas. She introduced me to the teachers. They seemed relaxed and not in the least ill at ease to have a stranger in the room. I learned that the Montessori principles were applied to the learning environment. Items the child could hold and manipulate filled the room. One tray held a husk of corn and tweezers. The child could squeeze the kernels off the cob with tweezers and drop them into a bowl. Another activity for the child involved a dropper with food coloring and a pitcher of water. Activities, I now recognized from Ben's OT experience, which were designed to increase fine motor strength and coordination. Puzzles, a birdcage with two birds fluttering, an aquarium, and a portable chalkboard provided a heavenly environment for curious children.

Nancy explained that the children were encouraged to pursue their natural talents, while the basics were also taught. The school operated with a contract system—a simple sheet of paper—where the child would accomplish tasks in core areas such as math and language arts and then the tasks would be individualized to the child's areas of strengths and weaknesses. The student–teacher ratio was ten to one, or less, most of the time.

"It's so quiet," I commented as various groups of kids sat down to work on projects together.

Nancy smiled. "Thank you. This is free-play time. But you have to understand that we're well into the school year and the children know the routine. We devote days and weeks to getting the children 'normalized' to the routine. Rights and responsibilities go hand in hand."

I watched as a child picked up a small broom and dustpan and started to sweep up the crumbs he'd left from his snack.

Nancy must have followed my eyes. "They can take as much as they want, but they have to eat what they take and clean up after themselves."

"Wow," was all I could say.

One of the teachers announced "Circle Time" and reminded those leaving for the day to check their drawers.

"Some of the children stay all day and some just for the morning. We're quite flexible," Nancy explained.

"But my son, Ben, who'll be entering kindergarten, would come every day, right?"

"Yes. We require kindergartners to attend school daily." She paused as we both watched the room's activities. "Tell me a little bit more about your son. You mentioned he's receiving speech therapy."

I took a breath. I wanted desperately for Ben to come here, but I didn't want to misrepresent the truth. This place seemed safe. No more kicks to the gut and not being able to tell me what happened.

I finally said, "He's a late bloomer. Just like his dad in so many ways. Late to talk, just like his father. But his speech is much improved, and he'll continue with speech therapy over the summer." I turned to meet Nancy's slightly unconvinced eyes. "This would be a wonderful place for my son." There must have been something in my voice, a quiet plea.

"You have to understand, we don't offer speech therapy here."

"Yes. I'll continue to have him in private sessions."

She met my eyes, and I tried not to blink. "I'll give you the enrollment papers to take home, then."

I filled them out, wrote a check, and returned them within a week.

* * *

IN MAY, WE SAID GOOD-BYE TO VIRGINIA, WHO FELT THAT Ben had made strides with social skills. She mentioned that he seemed to have some kind of "processing" problem. I wasn't sure what she meant. I asked John, and he shook his head. "He doesn't have anything wrong with his thought processes." He assumed she was referring to a mental illness such as schizophrenia. But Virginia hadn't said that specifically. In all, I felt gratitude toward her for accepting Ben and trying to make him feel a part of the group.

We also decided to take a vacation. It was long overdue, and John's job seemed fairly stable at the moment. John's parents lived in Estes Park, Colorado, a place of fond childhood memories for him and beautiful vistas that he'd missed seeing. Since I didn't particularly like flying, we drove for twenty-one hours across the country with the thought of taking the boys to "see America."

The night we arrived, my mother-in-law had made pizza for us, knowing the boys enjoyed it. Something inside me didn't feel right. I kept rubbing my stomach, complaining of a vague ache. I attributed it to the long two days in the car and the higher altitude.

Two hours later, curled into the fetal position, I sobbed with pain.

"It's okay, honey." I saw John's drawn face above mine. "I think you have appendicitis."

At first, his words didn't sink in. That meant surgery. An emergency. But I knew he was right. My hand slowly felt my right lower abdomen. The weight of my fingers was enough to make me scream.

"Yes. I know it is," I whispered. "Take me to the hospital. I can't stand it." I tried turning, lying flat on my back, but there was no relief from the deep cutting pain that made childbirth seem like a simple paper cut.

"Okay. Try to sit up."

I tried, but leaned heavily on John. "The boys will be okay?"

"Yeah, they'll be fine. My folks will take care of them."

I heard two little voices in the hallway. "Pete? Ben? Come in. It's okay."

Two little boys came in, blankets dragging on the floor. Peter was sucking his pacifier full force. Ben tried to give me his blanket.

"No. Not right now, honey. Mommy's okay. She's just got a really bad tummy ache. You're going to stay with Grandma and Grandpa, and I want you to listen to what they tell you. Okay?"

Two nods. Two pairs of eyes, one blue and one brown, stared back at me. I heard Peter start to cry and gently said, "Grandma and Grandpa will be here with you, honey."

I turned to Ben. "You're my big-boy. You take care of Peter for me and Daddy."

He nodded and moved closer to Peter.

A little while later, I managed to get in the car. John told me we were headed to Boulder, based on his mother's recommendation.

It was sleeting, and the sky had descended upon the road. We were driving through a white misty cloud that reminded me of a haunted house. The thin air coming into my body accentuated the pain, making me short of breath. My lungs were used to heavy, moist Midwest air. My gut twisted again, making me cry out. The pain came in waves, as if someone's hands were torturing me from inside. John slowed down as the visibility decreased. The road curved and sloped.

I felt a brief relief. "I know what hell is." I chuckled, and then grabbed my abdomen, wishing I hadn't.

John turned toward me. "Huh?"

I gasped. "I'm sure it could be worse, but right at this moment, it's about as bad as it gets. I'm in terrible pain. The goddamn road is knocking me all over the car. We seem to be sliding down a mountain that we can't even see. I'm hundreds of miles from home. I'm away from my kids. And there's a real chance I could die." I wiped a tear away. "I think God has handed me a load of shit."

* * *

WE FINALLY REACHED THE HOSPITAL. JOHN HELPED ME INSIDE, and I felt his strong arms supporting me. It struck me again how he was always a steady presence when things were bad. How he held me together. I'd forgotten.

A young ER technician sat in front of a triage screen and handed me some forms. I filled in the information with the exception of "weight" and put the clipboard through the slot.

"Just a minute." He scanned the form. "How much do you weigh?"

"A lot," I said. I figured a little sense of humor could go a long way at a time like this.

He stared at me through his designer frames. I had him pegged as a wannabe medical student with just enough training to make him dangerous. He didn't blink.

"Okay." I grimaced. I told him my weight, but shaved ten pounds off. There, I thought as I went to sit down. Another wave of pain slapped me into the chair.

"Why don't we just leave?" I asked John. "It's not so bad."

"No way. You're getting checked out." He picked up a magazine, which annoyed me.

"But I'm not supposed to get sick. And the boys. They don't know your folks that well. They'll be scared to death. You go back as soon as you can. Promise?"

John put the magazine down, placed his hand on mine, and stood as they called my name.

Several blood tests, an ultrasound, general anesthesia, and six hours later, I was minus one "hot" appendix. My father-in-law, John, and the boys came to see me the second day. John told me that Ben had done pretty well. It was my little Peter, soon to be three years old, who had screamed for his "Mama" and was inconsolable. All I could do was hug my boys and realize again how much being a mother made me capable of loving beyond anything I could have imagined.

* * *

AFTER OUR TRIP TO COLORADO, BEN WAS REASSESSED BY both Anju and Elizabeth. I'd grown to dread any kind of retesting since my experience with the university clinic. But the insurance company demanded it for continued services. Anju readministered the Clinical Evaluation of Language Fundamentals–Preschool (CELF-P) to check his receptive and expressive language skills, and tested his ability to speak intelligibly via the Goldman-Fristoe Test of Articulation. These were her original tests, and thus she could determine what sort of progress Ben was making by comparing the two points in time.

Anju's report summarized her findings:

Receptive language skills have increased almost 30 points, rating his receptive language skills from severely impaired to mildly impaired in 13 months. His Expressive Language Score, although increased slightly, is still severely impaired. His word recall and relating functional events, although not reflected on this test, have increased significantly. This child has come a long way from using only three dozen words expressively to relating to his parents when someone has hurt him or if his younger sibling needs help. His speech intelligibility or articulation has improved from 65% to 80%. Ben also performs receptively much better with visual cues.

I agreed with her assessment, and I sensed that the truth about Ben's functioning could be agreed upon by both the clinician and the parent. It didn't have to be separate impressions or realities.

Elizabeth administered the Peabody Developmental Motor Scales (PDMS) for a second time. Her report stated:

Ben's chronological age is 63 months; his fine motor age equivalent is 50 months, which indicates a 13-month delay. He was also tested with the PDMS on March 27. At that testing, Ben had presented with a 19-month fine motor delay. Therefore, he has made a six-month improvement developmentally in a three-month time span.

The insurance company approved continued therapy.

IN LATE SPRING, I NOTICED AN AD IN OUR LOCAL PAPER FROM a person offering in-home tutoring. The woman I spoke with had a pleasant, smooth voice. She told me she would be student teaching in special education in the fall. She'd gone back to school for a second degree in special ed and was about my age. Jamie was a single parent with a son who was also language delayed. Perhaps it was the slant of her face when she listened to me tell Ben's story, or the way her eyes registered the feelings I expressed, but I somehow knew Jamie's life hadn't been easy. The way I figured it, people who'd had a difficult life either grew hard or compassionate. Jamie had grown compassionate.

She agreed to come twice a week during the summer. I felt as if I were filling out a prescription for Ben for the three summer months: ST to continue twice weekly with OT once a week. At-home tutoring twice weekly.

The summer progressed with weeks of hard work and long trips to and from the children's clinic. The dog days of summer descended, and I kept a watchful eye for any more snakes that happened to want to visit. I'd pretty much healed from the surgery, but I had to constantly reassure Peter that I wasn't sick and wouldn't leave him. I attended my second writers' conference at the university and gradually felt in tune with the vocabulary the workshop leader used. I learned even more this time around, finally understanding proportion, revising texts, and the "ah ha!" moments in stories. It was an oasis of self in the summer of mothering and therapy.

Jamie had faithfully come for the past few months, working to reinforce preschool concepts with Ben—everything from the alphabet and counting, to colors and shapes. On my way to do laundry, I'd glance at the table in the basement where she and Ben would be working. Jamie's warm brown eyes would search Ben's face. She'd encourage him. Wait a few seconds. Ask another question, leading him to find the answer. Rather than frustrate him, she knew when to step in.

On one August day, after answering a knock at the door, I called to Ben that Jamie was here.

"No work." He didn't turn around, but continued to concentrate on his PlayStation video game. He'd started playing games a few months earlier that were years above his age level. His thumb and fingers flew on the buttons as he watched the screen. I was proud of his expertise, and these silly games gave me evidence of his ability to think, react, and process information—at least visual information. And it made him feel good. He could see his points increasing, the game moving to the next level of play, and he received immediate feedback on just how well he did.

I pursed my lips, slightly annoyed. Jamie stood in the kitchen, patiently waiting, her tank top and shorts looking moist from the outside heat. Short black hair framed her round, pleasant face, and I offered her some water. Ben hadn't stopped playing, despite two more insistent instructions that he put the game up.

"Just a second," I said to Jamie.

I walked into the living room and whispered into Ben's ear, "You will stop right now. You will go with Jamie to the basement."

"I don't want." He started to cry. "I sick of work." His chubby fingers wiped the tears from his eyes.

I didn't know what to do. I wasn't sure how to separate age-appropriate rebellion from a child's plea that he was tired. A part of me was glad to see it. It was so normal.

"Ben, you've got to. Jamie is waiting." I glanced at the kitchen and noticed that Jamie had almost finished her water. Although he'd been a little resistant at times with Anju, this was the first time he'd voiced outright refusal to work.

"Ben!" My voice was firm.

"No!" The tears stopped. His eyebrows furrowed, and his mouth took on a stubborn set.

"Ben, downstairs now!" I started to walk away, hoping he'd follow.

Jamie said softly, "It's okay. Maybe we should reschedule."

I thought about it. Ben's curly head was still fixed at the TV screen, although the game was off. If I allowed him to do this, I would be setting a precedent.

"Ben, I'm going to count to three, and you need to be heading down those stairs by the time I get to three." I took a breath, hop-

ing Peter wouldn't wake up from his nap amid all the sound.
"One."

Ben stood up, crying again.

"Two."

He started to walk to the kitchen.

"Three."

He was at the basement door.

I walked up to him. "Thank you, Ben. I know you're tired. I
know it's hard." I pulled him toward me and held him in my
arms.

He wiped his face one more time, and followed Jamie's petite
frame down the stairs. Once he got started, Jamie told me he did
well in the session.

After that, I cut back on the tutoring until after school started.
Ben had told me what he needed. He was a person in his own
right, and I respected that. He didn't understand the urgency of
what he needed. He didn't know what the tests said or how delayed he was. All he knew was that he was tired and just wanted
to play.

Inside my mind, the purple water had changed from a smooth
silent flow to choppy, frothy hits against the boat that held Ben
and me. We weren't moving, or so it seemed. The hours of therapy had made only marginal improvements in my son. Expression, his major problem, or so I thought at the time, had only
slightly improved.

Over the summer, we'd found out Ben needed glasses for far-
sightedness. A pediatric optometrist who'd examined his eyes
also wanted to monitor his visual tracking. She suspected that
since he wasn't reading yet, his eyes just might not have been exercised enough. Another problem. Another difficulty to keep on
top of.

Sometimes at night, I envisioned running away. Getting into
my car and just driving. I knew I never would. But the bittersweet memory of all the freedom I enjoyed while single morphed
into a romanticized notion of how great it would be not to have

to deal with this, even for a little while. The guilt that followed such thoughts reinforced my belief that I fell far short of the images of mother on screen and television. I should be cheering Ben on, getting those pompons lifted high with Tony the Tiger chants of "you're doing gerrrr—ate." But I was so tired. Shitty Mother.

Although I had a history of being technologically resistant, I'd signed up with a popular Internet service and could now e-mail Rosa and my sisters. I felt more connected with others, up to a point. I could describe how Ben was doing and what funny new things Peter did, but sometimes I longed for more human contact, to be able to sit across from Rosa at a restaurant lunch table. And I worried about wearing her and my family out emotionally. In some ways, I felt more isolated.

John and I were in survivor mode. He worked in one city, we lived in another, and now the kids would be going to school in a third. I envisioned a fragmented life inside a car for the upcoming year. Still, knowing the Montessori school was a wonderful place for a child, I braced myself for Ben's entrance into kindergarten.

CHAPTER EIGHT

First Impressions

"IT'S OKAY, BEN. JUST RELAX."

"Nobody mean?"

"Of course not. This is a fun, fun place to be. I know it's your first day here, and it's okay to be nervous. But please, I tell you the truth. This is a good school." I tried to steer the car while continually glancing at Ben.

His little body was rigid. He hardly moved in the car as we sped down the highway toward school. A few weeks earlier, he'd fallen again, cutting his right temple area a good half inch and requiring stitches. The cut had healed nicely, now only a pink reminder of his tripping over a kitchen chair on a hot summer evening.

"You pick up?" His voice was low and flat.

"I'll pick you up in just a short time." I tried to remember to speak slowly to Ben, especially when he was anxious. "You'll have so much fun today."

His brown eyes peered through his round glasses. His hair was curly and light brown with blond highlights. At home, when he laughed, it made me want to laugh right along with him. That image was vastly different from the boy sitting next to me.

"I'll bet you'll sing songs and meet new friends. See that white barn? That'll be the sign that we're almost to school. It'll be okay, Ben."

His face was pale. He'd refused to eat breakfast and with his sensitive gag reflex, I didn't push it.

I looked at Ben again. He was desperately trying not to cry. "You know what? Tomorrow, Peter will be right next door to you. You'll need to check on your little brother to make sure he's okay."

John and I decided to enroll Peter, who just turned three, in the school as well. I worried that he was a bit too young—he'd be one of the younger kids in the classroom—but his verbal skills were solid, his ability to follow directions was sound, and I thought it'd be a good place for him to grow. We were still fighting intermittent ear infections, and I hoped they would subside soon. The pacifier was still used at home as a security device, but I thought that maybe with peer interactions, Peter would lose interest in it.

Peter was in a different preschool program with fewer and, overall, younger children than Ben's. But it was in a room right next door to Ben's and so the two brothers could see each other on the playground and throughout the day. The first two weeks were for normalization—the kids learning the routine. Ben and Peter's schedules were slightly different during orientation to the school, one going in the morning and the other in the afternoon. I would soon be making at least two round trips to the school per day, which translated to two or three hours on the road.

Ben's eyes opened a bit, and I saw a hint of a grin. "Peedar here?"

"Yep. Tomorrow."

I turned into the school parking lot. Parents were encouraged to drop their children off in the car line where the teachers waited—complete with umbrellas when it rained. I figured I could start tomorrow. After all, it was his first day of kindergarten.

I parked the car, went around to help Ben out, and took his hand. "Let's go inside and see Miss Mary." Mary was Ben's teacher, and I'd met her when I'd brought Ben to school last week to have a look around.

I saw Mary greeting other children, opening her arms wide to herd them through the classroom door. She reminded me of a mama Teddy Bear, her childlike face and big smile welcoming each one. Through her poised gestures and even voice tones, gentleness emanated from her. Children who knew her came up to her for hugs and to show her their new backpacks and lunch-boxes. Her casual shorts and T-shirt told me she was there to paint, dig, and play alongside the kids.

"Here's Ben," I said, feeling almost as scared as Ben.

"Hi, Ben." Her voice was incredibly soft.

"He's a little nervous," I said.

Ben's eyes dropped to the floor. "Hi."

"Let's get your jacket hung up," Mary said. She looked at him quizzically, with a speck of worry in her eyes.

I hated first impressions. I wanted to pull her aside and say, "Ben really isn't like this. He laughs all the time. He's like a regular kid at home when he's relaxed."

But I watched as he stiffly stood there, hardly moving, looking at the floor in silence as I went ahead and hung his jacket up for him.

"Let's go start the day, Ben." Mary slowly reached out and offered her hand to him. After a glance my way, he took it and walked into the classroom.

"Bye, Benny," I said softly.

JUST OFF THE MAIN STREET OF OUR SMALL TOWN, ON THE outside of a storefront window, a wooden cutout of a hand proudly stood like a giant High Five. In the middle of the two-foot tall sign, it said, "Palm Reading and Tarot Cards." It beckoned the tourists and the locals. And today, it beckoned me.

I'd just finished breakfast with Bridget, who'd declined my offer to accompany me to see Halley, the psychic. Perhaps that

was for the best. I'd found I had limited energy to be around people. To keep the smiles going. I needed the sweet isolation of
being alone. The boys had started their regular school schedules a
few weeks earlier, and I found I had a couple of hours in the
morning to myself. Both boys seemed to be adjusting well to the
new school, and I noticed Ben's anxiety seemed less than when he
was at Virginia's preschool. They liked knowing the other one
was right next door.

During my two previous visits to the psychic—I'd come with
John the first time, and Rosa once when she was visiting from
Chicago—I'd been impressed with Halley's ability to tell me
about myself. Present and future. Halley had looked at John's
outstretched hand and told him he was a healer. That he had
three "spirit guides" around him. Her description of Rosa's relationship with her husband was dead-on accurate. What the psychic didn't tell me, but I knew for myself, was that my friendship
with Rosa was now very fragile. I could sense her impatience and
frustration with my negativity about life. I couldn't help it or
seem to change. Yet I grieved the special closeness we'd shared for
so many years, and I didn't laugh much anymore.

I always felt eerily wanton when I came to the psychic's door. I
felt I was rejecting faith and God by short-circuiting the usual
route of prayer and candle lighting, choosing instead to be fed via
the astrological pipeline for a quick and dirty 30-minute fix-for-
the-future.

That's not to say that Halley was cutting open roosters and
doing a voodoo number inside her little shop. A poster of Jesus
adorned an inside door and self-help books—okay, with a few
tarot and psychic channeling-type paperbacks—lined the walls.
Two pastel etchings of Native American Indians sat in black
frames, rainbow-colored feathers sprouting from their headbands.
Halley had told me during my last reading that they were her
spirit guides. Somehow it made sense. The wicker furniture was
slightly uncomfortable, and I wondered what I would be told this
time.

I waited until the other customers exited. Halley was always busy, even during the week when there weren't as many tourists. She'd curled her shoulder-length blond hair today. Around the neckline of her turquoise pantsuit, small wooden beads rustled gently as she moved her stout figure through her doorway and into her chair. Instead of her reading palms, I pictured her at home with grandkids making tie-dyed T-shirts.

"I've read you before, haven't I?" Her blue eyes studied me, and the slight nasal stuffiness to her voice was oddly soft and comforting.

"Yes."

She got a tissue to wipe the perspiration off my right hand. Her hand was firm as it held mine, but movement wasn't constricted. The sureness of her touch helped me calm down. "You have two children." She squinted down at my hand, turning it slightly. "But I see a third."

I chuckled. "No, that's not possible." John and I had decided against having any more children. The decision came as another loss for me. I'd always wanted three children. Perhaps because my family of origin had had three kids. I also felt that a third would reduce the comparisons between Ben and Pete. But if John's language difficulties had somehow been handed down to Ben and made more pronounced due to my difficult pregnancy, I couldn't—wouldn't—want to take such a risk with a third child. Maggie, the woman from the university clinic whose child had been misdiagnosed, came to mind. I knew the same fear as she had about tempting fate with another child.

I blinked quickly and leaned forward as Halley continued.

"I see three inheritance lines. You have a very clean lifeline. You've been on a lot of medicine lately."

It was true. I'd needed antibiotics recently. Then I wondered who the inheritances would come from. Guiltily, I removed those thoughts from my head.

"I see recognition." She pointed to my hand with the tip of a pencil. "See here. Those stars in your hand. Recognition."

"You have met your soul mate in your husband. You have a very strong bond and are loyal to each other. You're stubborn and can have a temper. You like good quality things."

Those things were all accurate. She went on to tell me things I knew about myself. Things I knew but didn't like to admit to myself. Much of what she told me was the same as the previous two times. High marks for consistency.

She'd pulled out the tarot cards and asked me to cut the deck several times, and then to select ten cards. She told me about someone undermining me or having jealous feelings toward me. I had no clue as to whom this might be.

She told me that John and I knew each other in a former life, probably in an agrarian time in Europe. She told me about our tight finances. About another change in the future, perhaps with John's job.

I said haltingly, "My little boy. Could you tell me about my little boy? He has trouble talking." I struggled to keep my voice strong. "Will he be okay?"

"What's his birth date?"

I told her and watched as she scribbled down the month, date, and year.

"Oh, he's an old soul. Very old. You know, Moses couldn't talk either."

I stared at her, unsure what to say.

"You know, that just came to me." She blinked and seemed surprised. "About Moses." She bent down and reshuffled the cards. "Pick three."

She leaned over the cards I'd chosen. "It's going to be rough. Yes."

She grabbed the paper with his birth date again. Then she looked back at the cards.

I wiped my hands again on the tissue.

Her head came up slowly and her brow was wrinkled. "But I show he's going to be okay."

I let out a sigh and collected my purse. "Thank you."

"Let me give you a hug," she said, standing up. "You know Jesus loves you, and with His light in our lives, anything is possible."

I left the shop and headed for my car. As I walked, a peace came over me. My breathing came more easily, and in the back of my mind, I clung to those words, "He's going to be okay."

SCHOOL PROGRESSED, AND AS THE WEATHER BECAME COLDER, Ben warmed to his new school. He developed his first friendship with a small boy named Frank. Frank, it seemed, got into trouble quite frequently, and had a shaky ability to stay on task. But the fact that Ben had someone to call a friend meant a lot to him.

Originally, Ben was signed up for morning-only kindergarten. Mary stopped me one November day to let me know that most kindergartners at the school attended four and a half days per week. I promptly changed his schedule. The change, however, meant that it would be next to impossible to continue with Anju since the school and Anju were in different cities, one on each side of our town. We'd already halted OT and seeing Elizabeth for the time being. Our decision was based on the gains he'd made—he showed only a mild delay in fine motor skills—and the fact that he'd be getting lots of fine motor activities in his days at school.

But because of expressive needs, I kept him in speech therapy for as long as I could. I hated the thought of saying good-bye to Anju. I'd crocheted a blanket for her, making it out of a soft wool yarn in various shades of purple, red, and gold. I wanted her to know how grateful I was, how this afghan that I hoped would bring her comfort was a gift from my heart. Anju and Elizabeth meant more to me than just my son's therapists. They were my support system.

But logistically, the therapy couldn't continue. Even on Ben's half day, I'd drive over an hour to reach Anju's office, and Ben was totally exhausted by the time we got home. So on December 21, we saw Anju for the last time. Her discharge summary read:

Final session. Subjective: Mom reports he is very verbal at home and school. Objective: He's made significant improvement processing information using concepts like if, before and after. Ben uses descriptive language well in structured activities, e.g., "It is animal, has long neck." Ben is problem solving quite well for his age. He can sequence events/activities with 80% accuracy and verbalize these without any difficulty. Action: Ben has made excellent gains in speech and language. His motivation and parental involvement are major contributors. Plan: Ben will be attending full day school and hence, he will not be attending ST here. Continue with concepts learned, sequencing, and use of final consonants, particularly t and s, were emphasized for home programming.

I lingered at the receptionist's desk, hugged Anju, feeling her slight frame next to my generously padded one. I was leaving something very important behind. I don't think Ben fully understood that this was his last visit with Anju. He shyly hugged her and smiled. They'd been through a lot together. As with my exit from the university clinic, I didn't have a plan in mind.

As we left the therapy offices, I asked Ben to push the down button on the elevator, pretended to smile, and couldn't shake the old fear that started to grow again inside me with the same question: What are you going to do now?

I WAS CUTTING BEN'S FINGERNAILS ONE DAY AND NOTICED ripped skin on the sides.

"Benny, don't do that!" I held up his fingers and kissed them.

He shrugged his shoulders and looked at his nails. "I know."

I looked at the ends, which were almost bloody. "It's okay. Try not to be nervous, okay? It's all right. Miss Mary is really nice, right?"

He nodded.

"And Frank is your friend, right?"

Ben smiled.

I wrapped my arms around him. "Please try not to do this." I cut the loose pieces of skin off and kissed his hands again. He went into the living room to watch TV, his head bent low as he looked at his hands.

The phone rang and it was Bridget. Her two sons and Ben and Pete still enjoyed play dates together. I told her I wasn't sure what to do with Ben, that I knew he still needed speech therapy. She told me about a computer program called Fast ForWord that was supposed to help kids' speech. When I pressed her with questions, however, she told me she didn't know very much about it. But there was also a speech therapist that Bridget knew who would come to the house. It would be a private pay or out-of-pocket arrangement. The hourly charge seemed competitive. Bridget had used the therapist with her son and said she had been pleased with her services.

Once again, Bridget had come through with valuable information. Most friends share tips on where to shop. We gave each other tips on therapists and how to stimulate speech skills. We knew not to ask too much of the friendship. But in an unspoken way, we provided a safety net for one another, giving solace during those times when our sons' problems overwhelmed us.

A couple of days later, I called Casey, the private speech therapist, and she agreed to see Ben at the house every other week. I hoped she'd give me things to do with him on the weeks she didn't come. Even with that arrangement, I calculated the cost and realized the cars would have to go another year or two.

About this time, I also started to attend a writers' group once a month. One of the participants I'd met at the writers' conference over the summer had sponsored my membership in the group that screened folks wishing to join. The group had been around for years and tried to keep membership to about a dozen with seven or eight representing a well-attended meeting. Members hosted in their homes on a rotating basis. Nothing was taken home. All the business—critiquing others' work—was done right then and there.

The membership was eclectic and exceptional. A mystery writer working on her fourth novel. A Christian writer who also enjoyed writing "whodunits." An essayist who had a talent for making the banal in life interesting. Several members had their masters in fine arts and wrote short stories that ranged from literary pieces to medieval Roman fantasies. They accepted me, tentatively at first, then as I joined in the discussions, with camaraderie. I felt I'd found a second home.

ALSO IN THE EARLY WINTER MONTHS, WE LEARNED THE GOOD news that John would be able to take the kids to the Montessori school in the mornings. The bad news was that he would be starting a new job in the same city as the boys' school. Again, we weren't quite sure what had happened. There were pressures to keep the patient billings up. Clashes over the lack of marketing for the adolescent inpatient unit he'd opened. Big things. Small things. Important things. The change had taken us by surprise. He'd requested the remainder of his vacation over the Christmas break, and I could see that he was bored, nervous, and melancholy at times. I was trying to be positive, which didn't come naturally to me.

We'd taken the Christmas tree out of the barn and pulled out the decorations. The boys were in charge of the unbreakable ones, like the construction paper reindeer with pipe-cleaner whiskers, and the plastic figures with loops of string instead of wire hooks.

"It'll help a lot that you'll take the kids to school." I stooped to help Peter unwrap an angel.

"Thanks." John sorted through a box of Christmas lights.

"It might be a real blessing in disguise," I said. "Plus, as the inpatient medical director, you'll be able to use your skills in consult-liaison work and geriatrics."

John began to wind the lights around the tree. "I guess so."

"It's much better than moving to Fort Wayne. Don't you think?"

"Yes, I think so," he said absently, connecting two sets of lights.

I continued to watch him in silence. He'd also been offered a job in Fort Wayne, Indiana, with a large medical center, about three hours north of where we lived. We'd thought long and hard about what to do. I'd gotten used to the freedom and privacy I had in the country. If I wanted to cut John's hair on the deck in the middle of a Sunday morning, I could. If I yelled loudly to get the boys' attention, I didn't have to worry about disturbing any neighbors.

But we considered what a larger city would mean for the boys. I wondered if closer playmates would be good for them. They'd have more options for private schools and easier access to speech services. I tried to see it from their perspective. They loved this place and their dogs. We'd have to give a couple of the dogs away if we moved. Ben and Peter wouldn't understand that. Ben was a child who loved structure and predictability. I worried that the change would traumatize him. And I knew my boys were safe here. No cars or streets to navigate. Fishing and swimming in our backyard. I realized how much I'd be giving up.

So when a job in the city to the east of us came up, the same city where the kids went to school, John accepted it. It meant we didn't have to relocate, and John's commute would actually be easier. He would be the inpatient medical director of the psychiatric unit, which housed adults only. No more treating children or adolescents. John would be accountable to two institutions; the community hospital that oversaw the unit, and the mental health center that provided the psychiatrists to treat the patients. There was no question: Between the decline in accessible mental health services and the fact that he would now have two employers, John's dream of returning to a private practice and treating children and adolescents faded further away.

JANUARY IN INDIANA PROVIDED ME WITH CHEAP THRILLS, especially when getting up the hill to our house. Each day the weather could be treacherous with snow or ice, or just cold. Today it was just cold. When I picked the kids up, I tightened up a bit, never quite sure if Ben would get into the car happy or upset about something that had happened. I worried that I'd be found out, that they'd say Ben couldn't make it there. Some of Ben's classmates were extraordinarily bright.

But today as I pulled up, I saw Mary smiling brightly. I smiled back, leaning over to greet her at the car door.

Ben jumped into the backseat of the car. I'd picked Peter up earlier in the day and he was resting in his car seat next to Ben, listening to every word of the conversation.

"I have to tell you," Mary started. "Ben is reading!"

"What?" I laughed giddily.

"He didn't seem to be getting the phonic sounds, so I decided to try him on some sight-reading books and he's just taking off!" She put her hand on her chest, trying not to cry. "It's wonderful."

I blinked rapidly. "That's great!" I turned around to pat Ben on his leg. He smiled proudly. "I read. It easy."

Mary glanced at the waiting cars behind us and hurried on with her explanation, "I can show you the books I'm using. You may want to buy some for home. It's a neat reading series called 'Key Words Reading Scheme' from a publisher called Ladybird Books. Key words are highlighted and repeated on each page. Simple words like 'I,' 'like,' 'dog,' and 'is.' It's not phonetically based. Instead, the child memorizes the words by 'sight.'" Mary took a deep breath. "Ben did wonderfully well."

I couldn't stop smiling. "That's so terrific. Of course, I'd like to have some at home. I'll stop by tomorrow. That's a great idea."

Mary leaned inside for a moment and said to Ben, "We read *Look at This* today, didn't we, Ben? A whole book."

Ben wiggled in his seat, so happy and so proud. "Tomorrow, read again?"

"Yes, sir." Mary waved at all of us and stepped away.

I said, "Thank you, Mary. Thank you so much."

She nodded, and her eyes welled up with tears. "Bye, Ben. See you tomorrow."

I pulled my van back on the highway, feeling a release in my stomach. I looked in the rearview mirror at Ben. "Mommy is so proud of you, Ben. You're reading! That's absolutely fantastic."

"We get chicken and French fries?" Ben asked.

"Can we get? You betcha." I laughed. "How about you, Pete? Are you hungry?"

My blond-haired boy looked back at me with his blue eyes and nodded. "A toy, too!"

IN MID-FEBRUARY, THE MONTESSORI SCHOOL TOOK THE kindergarten students to the elementary school building to be introduced to the first grade teachers and classroom. I'd received the notice and tried to explain it to Ben one more time as we drove to school that day.

"I go there now?"

"No. You'll go just to visit for the day."

"I still with Miss Mary?"

"Yes, Ben."

"Miss Mary still teach me?"

"Yes. You're just going to see where you'll be next year."

Ben started to say something and stopped. I don't think he quite got it. "You're just going for a visit."

Mary called me later that night. Luckily, John was home, and I took the call on the basement extension. "Ben was pretty scared today."

"You mean when he visited the first grade?"

"Yes. He just kept repeating that he wanted to go back to kindergarten."

"I understand. I've seen Ben when he's like that. I know the ruminations can put people off. He can really get stuck on something." My hand pulled the hair back from my forehead. The impression the other teachers got of him must have been horrendous. I'd seen those times when he obsessed on something due to anxiety. I hadn't anticipated the visit would be such a big deal for him, but I knew he'd finally grown comfortable in kindergarten and felt secure. That had been threatened when he thought he was leaving it and Mary. The threat had been too much for him to handle. In her tactful sweet way, she was telling me that Ben had had a major meltdown.

"Well," Mary said and hesitated. I held my breath and knew something was coming. She continued, "Miss Rice, the first-grade teacher, feels that after next year this school may not be the best place for Ben. She thinks first grade would probably be okay since the children are still in one classroom, but after that . . ."

An alarm started going off in my head. "I'm not sure what you mean."

"It's just that we may not be able to meet Ben's needs. And we can't offer Ben speech services here."

"I've arranged for private therapy at home. The therapist comes here to work with him."

"Yes, but there are other factors. We're not designed to really meet the needs of children with the learning difficulties that Ben might have."

"I see."

"We just want to be able to meet the student's needs. Miss Rice feels that we possibly wouldn't be able to do that with Ben. But we can wait and see. I'm just saying that it's a possibility."

"Oh." A brief silence. "But he's sight-reading. I know he can do it."

"I think so, too. And things can change a lot in a year. He's made good progress. I just wanted to let you know what happened today."

"Yes. Thanks. I'll discuss this with my husband. You're saying that he won't be able to go there after next year?"

"No. We just wanted to let you know that it's a possibility." Her voice softened. "He seemed really scared. He wasn't able to focus, and we finally had to take him back to the kindergarten room."

I crossed my legs. "I understand. Thanks for calling."

After I hung up, I sat in the basement and noticed my hands shaking. It was such a great school. It had offered me security as well. I didn't have to worry about testing and misdiagnoses and kids making fun of him. Peter was thriving as well, really blossoming under the direction of his teachers and the free open learning environment.

My stomach started to churn. I remembered that the boys and John must be finished with dinner. I put my face in my hands and at that moment, I didn't know what to do. Why was it so difficult for Ben to talk? Why, when he could remember words and read, could he not utter a normal sentence? I thought that since he was sight-reading, he was on the right path. That they'd keep him there for sure.

I wheeled the chair away from the phone and slammed myself up to the roll-top desk. Anger. Why couldn't he hold it together? I'd reassured him. Maybe I should have been there with him. I just hadn't done enough.

And why did the school put so much weight on one meeting? The snapshot effect again. Mary knew he wasn't normally like that. Miss Rice didn't know him, granted, but couldn't she take Mary's word that this little boy was just scared out of his mind?

I stood up, almost tripping over the legs of the chair. A despair floated in the air around me, like a fog hanging thick above the purple water, and I inhaled deeply.

I'D RECEIVED AN ADVERTISEMENT IN THE MAIL—I'M NOT SURE how our name and address were found—on a software program called Earobics, which was distributed through a company called Cognitive Concepts. The brochure said the software cost less than a hundred dollars and targeted auditory discrimination, memory, and other listening skills. I carefully put the brochure aside. I remembered the other program that Bridget had mentioned called Fast ForWord. I'd found out that it cost hundreds of dollars and required a trained provider to administer.

I didn't get it. The two programs sounded like they targeted the same areas, but differed vastly in the cost, accessibility, and intensity. I could do Earobics myself. No provider was necessary. I was desperate to try anything. After years of traditional speech therapy, first at the university clinic and now with Anju, Ben was marginally more expressive. Maybe this software could help him. The urgency to do more prompted me to get more information.

Casey, the private speech therapist, came faithfully on her appointed day, always a half hour late. Her only available session was during the "Real Adventures of Johnny Quest" on the Cartoon Network, Ben's favorite show. So I'd slip a tape into the machine and record it for him. He rarely resisted going downstairs with Casey, and once he got started, he worked hard.

One afternoon, I stopped Casey. "Have you heard of Fast For-Word?"

"A little." She paused. "I know that to become a provider, I'd have to go to New York, and the costs are too much for me to handle right now."

"I see."

"And I wonder how it works. I've read some of the literature. It sounds good, but it's just too hard for me to get certified. I've also heard it's expensive and takes an hour and a half every day, five days a week." She shrugged her shoulders. "They're sure making some big claims on what it does."

"What about Earobics? Have you heard of that?"

"Just a bit. I'm not too familiar with that either."

I thanked her for the information before she and Ben started their work together.

A few days later, I called a mom whose name and number I'd gotten through a mutual friend. The friend had told me this person had used Fast ForWord with her daughter. I introduced myself, and she said she'd be happy to tell me about Fast ForWord, but had to pick up her little girl in a few minutes.

"What is Fast ForWord?" I started.

"It's a series of computer 'games,' but they're more than games. It trains the child to—I don't know—process, identify sounds. We did it as a home site."

My voice became more urgent. "Home site. You mean you did it at home? They let you do that?"

"Yes—well, they screen you. We did it at home every day, an hour and a half every day for six weeks."

"Did it help your child?"

A short hesitation. "Yes, I think so."

"Did it help her speech?"

"A little. We followed up with some of the Lindamood-Bell programs. I think that's what really helped my daughter. She gets As in spelling now."

"Lindamood-Bell?" I clutched the phone. I reminded myself of a bloodhound on the scent of a fresh new trail.

"It's hard to explain. It's called the LiPS Program. The traditional idea of grouping consonants and vowels is kind of thrown out the window, and the child learns the sounds by the sensation and feelings of the sounds. Phonemic awareness, I think it's called. I did that with her myself, too. I took training through a lady in Indianapolis. I'm not sure if she still does it. It's not that hard to do. I'd be willing to show you the materials you'd need."

She went on to explain more about Fast ForWord and told me that her provider was the head of a large private clinic that offered rehabilitative services for adults and children. She told me the cost, and I swallowed hard. She wasn't familiar with Earobics.

We chatted a bit more, and I asked her if I could call her again, later if need be, and she said yes. She had been so generous to a stranger. Our only link was the fact that we were mothers of children who struggled.

I DECIDED TO ORDER THE EAROBICS STEP 1 PROGRAM FIRST. With the logistic differences between the two programs, I thought it was worth checking out. When it came, John downloaded it into the computer, and I had Ben attempt to play. There were six games, with different tasks, all of which targeted listening skills. There was one called "Rhyme Time" with Bog Frog, a deep-voiced swamp frog whose instructions dealt with rhyming

and adding louder and louder background noise as the child progressed. There was absolutely no way Ben could do this game.
His frustration escalated with each attempt. The other games
were also next to impossible for him. After a week, although the
program was a good one, I knew my son wasn't ready for it.

After discussing all that I had discovered with John—the information from the woman whose daughter had used Fast For-
Word, Casey's input, and Ben's reaction to Earobics Step 1—we
decided to call the private clinic to find out more about Fast For-
Word. Ben was nearing the end of kindergarten, and Mary had
told me he'd attained all the skills necessary to advance to first
grade. His speech was still severely delayed and no one needed to
tell me that, although he was being promoted, he needed a lot of
remediation.

My fingers shook as I dialed the private clinic's long distance
number. The receptionist picked up and told me that Gloria Lawson, the clinic's owner and director, wasn't in that day.

"Can you tell me if you allow people to do Fast ForWord at
home?"

"I don't make that determination. There are certain guidelines
for that. But I do know that we have set people up as home sites
in the past."

"Do you know if parents have been pleased with the program?"

"Oh, yes. I can tell you that. The pre- and post-test scores have
been amazing."

"When can I get my son in to see Ms. Lawson?"

"How about next Friday?"

"That'd be great." I gave her my name, address, and phone
number. "One more thing. Can you tell me a little about Ms.
Lawson's background? I mean, is she an SLP?"

"Sure. Yes, she's a speech-language pathologist with over thirty
years' experience in working with adults and children. She has a
master's degree and has earned her CCC-SLP or Certificate of
Clinical Competence in Speech-Language Pathology. We also
have two audiologists on staff who are also CCC in Audiology."

"Impressive."

"She's very good," the secretary's voice seemed to imply that she wouldn't be working for her if she weren't.

I hung up the phone and felt dazed. Maybe, just maybe, there was a flicker of hope. An answer out there for my son. My desperation had grown into an obsession that was eating at me, swallowing me, and at the same time, fueling me with enough energy to continue my search—to never stop believing in Ben. Something inside told me I was being thrown a lifesaver in the purple water.

CHAPTER NINE

Riddle Solved

I KEPT MY THOUGHTS TO MYSELF AS JOHN, BEN, AND I SPED north toward Indianapolis. It had been almost three years since the three of us had taken a similar drive to the university clinic where Ben had first been tested. I shook my head nearly imperceptibly. Three years and the puzzle still hung around us. This struggle was now as much about me as about Ben. Sometimes I thought I'd grown too emotionally dependent on his progress or lack of progress, living a life contingent on my son's functioning. Obsessive Mom versus Shitty Mom.

We lived about two hours away from the private clinic. The clouds hung low and dark on the early summer day. Ben seemed content, and we'd let him bring his Game Boy with a couple of cartridges. He played for a while and then would look out the window. I turned around to look at my six-year-old little boy. "I love you, Ben."

His wonderful smile formed. "Love you. We there?"

"No. Not quite." I cleared my throat, thinking he already looked tired. "Ben, do your best today, okay? Just try really hard to answer their questions. It'll be like when you saw Anju."

He stared back at me, his eyes serious behind his round glasses. "Okay?"

He nodded, and I stroked his soft cheek before turning back around. My mind reached further into the past, and I nudged up to the window, closing out John's presence next to me. The echoes from eight years ago, voices, seemingly recent, filled my ears. A falling out with an important mentor at the university where I was studying for my Ph.D.

"Oblivion," he'd said. "You'll fade into oblivion if you don't interview with the right universities. If you don't make school a priority, that's all you'll have to look forward to."

I had made school a priority. But I owned a small home and was supporting myself. A part-time job as a long-term care consultant, and two grad assistantships allowed me to live and go to school. Still, I finished my degree in three years and was offered praise and encouragement by my professors.

After passing my final exams, I didn't interview with the top universities. In fact, I hadn't interviewed with any, choosing instead a job at a nearby hospital as a nurse researcher. I had my first date with John the day I turned my dissertation in.

I glanced at John's profile as he navigated the busy interstate, and then I retreated again to remember choices from the past. On this particular day, I'd never felt closer to that feeling of being totally forgotten by the world and wondering about all the "what ifs" of different paths offered to me. Oblivion, indeed.

Then I looked at John again, this time with gentle eyes, and thought how Ben and Pete had framed our entire relationship. How our struggles with Ben had challenged our marriage and us. We'd seen each other at our worst and our best.

"You know," I said, breaking the long silence, "I got my International Communication Association Membership directory the other day."

"Okay." He knew I'd brought it up for a reason.

"I saw the listings for each member, their names, an 'h' by their home phone numbers, an 'o' by their office numbers. Then it had all these 'fs.'" I giggled. "Do you know what I thought when I saw those 'fs'?"

John smiled. "What?"

"Friends. For God's sake, I thought it meant 'friends.' And I thought, 'Boy, do these people have a lot of friends.'" I broke out laughing. "That's how pathetically out of it I am. It took me a while to figure out that it meant 'fax.'"

"You're not out of it."

"Yes, I am. But that's okay. It's okay." I straightened up in my seat and lowered my voice. "Do you think they'll help Ben at this place?"

"Yes, I do."

I knew John didn't know, but at that moment, I needed to hear it and he loved me enough to say it.

BEN WAS IN HIS USUAL FIRST IMPRESSION MODE. EYES TAKING in everything. Expressive skills dropping even lower than normal. A voice becoming a whisper. Staying close to John and me. It tore at me that he was so scared, that he had to go through this again and again and again. I promised him a special lunch with Mommy and Daddy and encouraged him to try to relax. It would be all right.

The office was really quite nice. I felt like a seasoned critic of speech clinic offices. They'd made a partial enclosure for kids to play in that looked like a log cabin, complete with painted woodland animals darting in foliage. The inside enclosure was filled with a chalkboard and some kids' toys, a small table and chairs.

I sat with a clipboard balanced clumsily on my lap, answering a developmental history sheet. There was a sheet called "Parent Checklist." This form was different from the ones I'd filled out in the past in that it asked for my input on specific areas of Ben's behavior. It was on a five-point scale and instructed me to rate Ben in many expressive and receptive areas such as "his ability to pay attention; to follow instructions; to understand a familiar adult; and to express thoughts using oral language with parent, another child, and a non-familiar adult." I recognized a similar form that I'd given to Mary to complete from a teacher's perspective. I checked most of Ben's abilities in the low range.

Shortly after turning in the forms, a petite brunette woman in her late-fifties approached us, smiling. She stretched out her hand. "Hello, Mr. and Mrs. Thompson. I'm Gloria Lawson."

We stood and shook hands.

"This must be Ben." She turned slightly toward him.

Ben looked at the floor. I didn't hear him respond. "He's a little nervous."

Gloria narrowed her dark eyes, still gazing at Ben, then spoke to us. "What I'd like to do is talk first with the two of you and then take Ben for some tests."

There was that word. I'd grown almost phobic when the word "test" was uttered. But of course I knew there would be tests done this morning. Gloria got a staff person to come and sit with Ben. I explained that Daddy and I were going to talk to Gloria, and we'd return in a little while. "You stay here and play, okay, Ben?"

He nodded. The young staff woman smiled easily at Ben and coaxed him into looking at a book with her. I wondered how much of all this he understood.

Gloria escorted us into her office. A desk with a computer, complete with screen saver, wicker furniture, another desk with a child's-size chair and two adult-size plush chairs were arranged neatly in the room.

We told her the same information we'd shared with all the others—from the university clinic to the private speech therapist. I sounded like a tape recorder asked to push Play. The only difference was our input on the parent checklist. I hadn't realized until I read the checklist questions just how many times Ben said, "huh?" and "what?"

Thirty minutes into the interview with Gloria, there was a knock at the door. The staff member assigned to Ben poked her head in. "He's a bit upset. I was wondering if I could get him a soda from the machine." She looked at us. "If it's okay with Mom and Dad."

Gloria looked at us, and we nodded.

"Is he crying?" Gloria asked.

"He's okay. He's just missing his parents. I think a drink will help." The young woman glanced at us as if trying to communicate that Ben was okay.

"Should I go to him?" I asked.

"No. Let's try a drink first." Gloria seemed concerned and said to her staff person, "Let me know if he doesn't calm down."

"He likes root beer," I said to the woman before she left. I tried to concentrate on what Gloria was saying, thoughts of Ben interrupting my concentration.

When I felt an opening in the conversation, I asked, "Can you tell me a little about Fast ForWord?"

Her voice became stronger, the topic obviously one she felt excited about. "Fast ForWord Language or simply Fast ForWord is wonderful technology. I'm very enthused about this product, and I've been in this field for over thirty years as a speech-language pathologist. I've seen it change brain functioning—in some patients. At least, that's my opinion."

I opened my mouth. "Wow."

"I know." She spread her hands on the papers on her desk. "That's saying a lot."

"We'd be very interested in getting this for him as a home site. I spoke with a previous client of yours, and she mentioned that that was possible."

"I haven't done the tests with Ben directly yet. I want to make sure he'd benefit from the program. Let's take it one step at a time."

"How does this work?" John put his hand under his chin. I could read him in doctor mode. His body resonated with skepticism.

I was ready to say, "Sign us up. Halleluiah, amen, and praise the Lord."

Gloria said, "It's a series of computer games that are actually auditory training exercises. The speech the child gets is altered, modified, slowed down, so that the child, particularly one with a temporal processing problem, can 'hear it.' As the games progress, the speech is brought to a normal level. I have a demo set up in the other room, and we'll get to that in a minute. It's easier to show you. But for now, I want to get Ben in here and do the testing." She pushed her chair back and stood up.

John and I walked down the hallway and saw Ben sitting next to the young woman with a can of root beer in his hand. His nose was a bit red, but he wasn't crying. His whole face brightened when he saw us, and John went to sit next to him, patting his arm. "You're okay, little guy."

We explained to Ben that he needed to talk with Gloria now, and we'd wait here for him. He separated fairly easily and accompanied Gloria down the hallway.

During the next forty-five minutes, I couldn't sit still, concentrate, or even carry on a conversation with John. He was annoyingly calm, or so he appeared. We chatted aimlessly about his new job, which seemed to be going okay.

As the medical director of the acute inpatient psychiatric unit, he saw incredibly ill people. More so than ever before in his career. The state-run hospitals for the chronically mentally ill were under fire from the media for poor quality of care and issues surrounding patient rights. The state, in its wisdom, hadn't sought to deal with these issues directly or prepare adequate community support programs. It had instead begun discharging patients into society who were ill-equipped to deal with life. It seemed the only thing that benefited was the state's budget. Many of these poor souls—the lucky ones—ended up hospitalized on John's unit.

It all made me very sad and feeling very tired.

Finally, Gloria emerged from the back offices with Ben. He grinned a bit, but I could tell he was tired. Gloria had the look of one who had bad news to share and didn't know quite how to say it.

"I'd like to do the audiological tests on Ben now."

"Can we do it here?" I asked.

"Yes. We're all set up. I have an audiologist who will perform the testing. I'll walk you back to her area and then see you when you're finished."

The four of us went back into the office suite again and met the audiologist, a chubby woman with pictures of a toddler on her desk.

"Okay, Ben." She smiled and gently guided him into a sound-proof booth. He looked so small as he sat down in front of the window where the audiologist would face him. She was carrying an otoscope and bent down to check each ear. "Okay. The ear canals and eardrums look good. Now I need you to wear these headphones over your ears. Like this. Does that feel okay?" After Ben nodded, she checked to make sure the headphones covered his entire ear.

She closed the door to the booth and walked around to her control panel. "Okay, Ben. We're going to start now." Ben seemed to be going with the flow. As long as he knew we were close by, he was okay. John and I couldn't see Ben, but we could hear him. "First I'm going to do a hearing test, then a screening test for auditory processing."

"Processing?" I said.

"It's a test called the SCAN. It has three subtests. One has distorted words that he has to repeat. The second one has background noise with the words, and the third subtest gives him two words at once."

I raised my eyebrows.

She grinned. "It's not easy. I always ask students who come to observe to take the third test, and they always say, 'That's really hard.' Some can't do it."

She faced the window and Ben. Then she proceeded to do the peripheral hearing test to make sure his hearing wasn't impaired.

"His hearing's okay, right?" I asked.

She looked at her sheet. "Seems to be. Gloria will go over all the test results with you."

Her fingers flipped a switch allowing Ben to hear her say, "Okay, you're going to hear some words. Repeat them back to me as best you can."

His voice was thin and shaky. There were times of silence.

The audiologist flipped a switch. "Just repeat what you hear. You're doing fine."

"I'm not sure he knows what repeat means." I sat up straighter. "Tell him to 'say the words back to you.'"

"I give them instructions two times, and that's all I can do," she explained.

Another shaky answer. His voice sounded so weak and young.

After a few more minutes, they were done. She wrote the scores down, and again I sensed bad news.

She got up quickly and released Ben from the booth. "Good job, Ben."

John gave Ben a big hug and smiled at him. My stomach reminded me I hadn't eaten much, yet I felt sick. I wanted Gloria to tell me what all this meant and how Ben had done. And I wanted her to tell me *now*.

"Okay, let's take this to Gloria." The audiologist edged out of the cramped room, and we followed her back to Gloria's office.

Gloria was seated behind her desk and stood up to look at the audiological results. Her eyes again narrowed, and her mouth frowned. The audiologist pointed to the dots on a blue background score sheet. I stole a peek and couldn't help but notice the negative standard deviation rankings. Gloria shook her head, making eye contact with the other woman. "Go ahead on home. Thanks for coming in."

We also thanked the audiologist before she excused herself.

Gloria scooted her chair closer to her desk and waited for us to sit down. "Ben isn't processing sounds the way he should. He has a lot of distortions in the way he's hearing. I found evidence of this with the tests Ben and I did as well."

"Distortions?" I asked.

"Just a second." Gloria glanced at Ben. "I think it's okay to talk in front of him. I don't think at this point he'd understand most of it, anyway." She put some small stuffed animals on a table for him to play with.

She started again. "Okay. Based on these tests, I would say that

Ben, in addition to his language deficits, has an auditory process-ing disorder. Have either of you ever heard of it?"

We shook our heads.

"We did a hearing test on Ben, and we know his hearing is normal. But the way he's processing sounds isn't. My other tests indicate some real problems in not only expression, but also re-ceptive abilities. The SCAN test that he just had—it stands for Screening Test for Auditory Processing Disorders in Children—indicates he's two standard deviations below the norm. It's a screening device, and I used other tests as well."

I looked at John and then asked, "What exactly is an auditory processing disorder?"

Gloria nodded as if just getting started on a long explanation. "Auditory processing disorder, or APD, isn't well-defined in aca-demic circles right now. In fact, we have a lot to learn about APD. Some call it 'central deafness,' or compare it to dyslexia by labeling it 'dyslexia of the ear.' Others, in fact, are skeptical APD even exists. My working definition is a general lack of proper au-ditory perception and/or processing. A famous definition by Jack Katz, one of most noted scholars in this area, is 'what we do with what we hear.'"

She paused to let the information soak in. "Part of the problem in understanding APD is that kids can have varied 'clinical pre-sentations'—how they appear to the professional. Unlike other difficulties, there's no one profile that fits these children. For ex-ample, some have trouble with speech and others don't. Some have lots of trouble with background noise and some don't."

"Do they know what causes it?" I watched Ben's small head bent low, playing with the stuffed animals on the other side of the room.

"Again, there are theories or educated guesses, but familial ten-dency seems to be a prominent one right now. Some say chronic ear infections put a child at risk, or the auditory deprivation—the sounds they miss—that occurs because of the ear infection. Some say it has something to do with neuromaturational development. In other words, the child's neurological development in the area of auditory perception is delayed for some reason. Lots of theories right now. Very few things we can say with absolute certainty."

"So hearing is not impaired, per se? That's why Ben turns when he's spoken to and jumps at loud noises."

Gloria nodded slowly. "There can be hearing deficits along with auditory processing disorder, but in most cases I've seen, it's a matter of processing sounds efficiently."

"So the child usually has normal hearing, but he can't make sense of the sounds."

"In a very basic sense, that's correct."

"Why have we never heard of this before?" I faced John for a moment. "Have you ever heard of it?"

"No." He shook his head.

"I mean, John has a medical degree, and I have a healthcare background. You'd think we'd have come across it at some point in time."

Gloria straightened the pen set on her desk. "Many people have never heard of APD. Some clinicians lump it into other categories of learning or developmental difficulties and don't see it as a singular impairment. The presentation of the child can fool someone easily. It looks a lot like other things."

I sat there silently for a few seconds, letting it all sink in, thinking of the diagnoses that were inferred regarding Ben. John seemed dazed and now had Ben, who looked very tired, sitting on his lap.

I continued finally, "And that's why speaking slowly helps Ben so much? Because it allows him time to process the sounds?"

"Or modifies it to the point that he can 'hear' it. The Fast ForWord technology modifies sound so that the child can process it."

"Then, Fast ForWord can help this? How does it work?" I asked.

Gloria smiled. "It was developed through collaborative efforts from Rutgers University—Drs. Paula Tallal, Steve Miller, and

some others—and the University of California at San Francisco—
Drs. Michael Merzenich, William Jenkins, and other folks. They
decided to combine efforts and came up with this amazing technology. It's based on the principle that kids with language im-
pairments have defective acoustic signal reception. They figured
out that by using intensive adaptive exercise—"

I shook my head. "I'm sorry?" She was losing me.

Her face remained serious, her eyes intense. "It means that this
program changes as the child progresses. It adapts uniquely to
how the child performs. Automatically. And as it adapts, it becomes more challenging until that level is accomplished. With
each level, the modified voice transforms incrementally to normal
speech. The exercises must be played according to the schedule. If
you are set up as a home site, it's imperative that you keep to the
schedule of play—five days out of seven. That's critical."

"I understand. Will we be able to do it with Ben?" My eyes
pleaded with her.

"I'll be honest with you. I'd like to see Ben on the demo. I'm
not sure he'll be able to do the games."

I looked sharply at her.

She continued to watch Ben, her face again totally serious.
"There are some basic skills the child needs to have—be able to
use a mouse, follow directions, understand shapes, sizes and colors, and attend to the games." Gloria stood up. "Let's go into the
other room where my assistant in charge of Fast ForWord has it
set up and see if he's able to do it."

"Okay." My legs felt numb and unstable. What did she mean,
"able to do it"? Inside, I was screaming he *had* to do this. He was
scared today. All he needed was a chance. After three years of
wondering, here was the first real understanding of what had
been affecting Ben. I wasn't leaving until he'd been given the
chance to prove himself.

We sat at an oval metal table, and Ben put headphones on
again and sat down next to Teresa, another young woman, who
also put headphones on.

"This lady is my lifeline." Gloria gave the young woman's arm a playful shake. "She's my computer wiz. Helps with all the technical support for Fast ForWord and helps people who are doing it at home."

"We'd be very interested in that," I said again.

Gloria's face dropped slightly. "Let's see if he can do it."

The woman at the computer beside Ben checked for his ability to work the mouse by pointing and having him position the cursor where she indicated. He'd used a mouse before and quickly got used to it again. "Okay, listen, Ben."

Three squares showed up on the screen. An altered voice—a woman's voice that sounded distorted, slowed down in the slightest way—said, "The baby is crying. The baby is crying." One square had a baby smiling. One had a baby crying, and one showed a baby with a neutral expression.

The woman motioned to the mouth of the baby, and showed Ben how to move the mouse to the right square. His hand took over operation of the mouse, and the next voice prompt came. "The clown has a balloon." Pictures of a clown with a balloon, a clown with a flower, and a boy with a balloon appeared.

Ben clicked on the right picture immediately. Then another set of images appeared and the voice gave another prompt. Ben again clicked right away.

The woman nodded to Gloria. "He's getting it."

Gloria watched. She wasn't sure. "I'd like to see how much he can read. You mentioned he was sight-reading."

"Yes," John said.

The woman had finished enough of the demo games with Ben and had exited the program. He came to sit next to Gloria, across from us at a large table. Gloria pulled out a reader, scooted closer to Ben, and asked him to read what he could. He started and stopped, barely able to make out a few words. Then she pointed to a word.

"What's that, Ben?"

"The."

"What's this word?"

"Is." And so on. He was able to identify about ten words.

"Okay," Gloria finally conceded. Then she looked at her assistant, who nodded at Ben and said, "He could do it. He did pretty well."

I waited, fidgeting in my seat, unsure whether I should pull Snake-Killing Mom out and demand he be allowed to do the program, or get on my hands and knees and beg.

Gloria turned to John and me. "Okay. I think he'll be okay."

I exhaled, still feeling like a member of the Collective Mom, an outsider knocking at the door to services. "How do we set it up?"

"You'll need to sign a lease with Scientific Learning Corporation, which makes Fast ForWord products. This is good for a six-month period of time, but you'll actually be playing the exercises for six to nine weeks. Then, you'll return the software to my office. You'll also need a computer with a fast enough processor and enough memory. I'll give you a sheet that tells you what you'll need. And you'll need to be online."

"We're already online. I'm on AOL."

She shook her head. "No, you'll need a full-service provider. You'll need to set up an e-mail address, and I'll e-mail you after Ben completes the games each day. You'll also be downloading his data after he plays on a daily basis."

I looked at John, not understanding. We'd been at the clinic for hours and combined with the two-hour drive, I was exhausted and feeling definite overload. John nodded confidently. He had a knack for computer stuff. Gloria handed John a sheet that gave the Apple and IBM compatible requirements for the program.

"Do we have a computer that will do it?" I asked.

"No. We'll have to buy one."

Next, Gloria handed us the leasing contract for the software. It was less than a thousand dollars. Then she explained her fee as the certified provider. Today's testing wasn't included, but the post-testing, after the program was completed, would be. Add over two thousand dollars.

But less than ten minutes ago, I'd watched my son respond to an altered voice in a way I'd never seen him respond before. His little head had bobbed confidently as the pictures flashed by and the mouse clicked. John appeared to be leaving the decision up to me. His skepticism had been pushed aside in deference to my judgment. It was my call.

"I just have one question."

"Yes," Gloria said.

"Do you take Visa?"

GLORIA PROVIDED US WITH A DEMO DISK OF THE GAMES. HER assistant gave John a crash course in playing the games and how Ben's results were to be downloaded to Scientific Learning. Gloria repeated, her voice firm and serious, that the program had to be played five days out of seven for the full hour and a half. We had to follow the schedule. We could not skip any games.

I clutched my purse and the demo CD, murmuring, "Okay. Okay. I understand."

Gloria turned to me as we finally walked down the hallway to leave. "You know, a year ago, I didn't have this technology to offer you. It didn't exist."

"I'm very grateful that it does." I shook Gloria's hand and left.

We loaded Ben into the car, all of us feeling exhausted and hungry. On the way home, we stopped for an early dinner at one of those places that served breakfast all day.

"Have you ever heard of auditory processing disorder?"

"No," John said.

"I haven't either." I paused. "But doesn't it make sense? All the pieces make sense now. If he wasn't able to process sounds, how could he learn to talk? It isn't that he's not bright, is it?"

"It has nothing to do with intelligence. Cognition or intellect is separate. Just like how Ben is able to show affection and know when we're upset. That's something else. I think he has a real gift for reading emotions, and I know he's bright." His words carried a vindication.

I studied John for a moment and knew him well enough to detect relief and guarded hope. His face seemed younger, his carriage lighter—the information Gloria had shared had taken away some of the sadness from his eyes. His faith in his son had been affirmed.

I took a sip of water. "It explains a lot about his anxiety, that's for sure. I mean if you're hearing gibberish or just parts of messages, but speech is all around you, I think anyone would be anxious or shut down. I think Ben knew he wasn't getting it. Imagine how hard that must have been for him." I swallowed. The bombardment of emotions constricted my throat. I looked away from the table, trying to focus on the country memorabilia on the walls. Trying to calm down. "But why didn't anyone even mention auditory processing before now? Why did it take three years to find this out?"

"I don't know. Like Gloria said, not many people know about it. I'm just glad we know now." He ruffled Ben's hair, interrupting Ben's feast of pancakes and bacon.

"I don't have a clue what she was talking about, as far as the computer stuff and the full-service provider. Do you get it?"

"Yeah. It's not that big a deal."

"It is to me. You'll take care of all of it?"

"Of course."

"So, let me get what Gloria said straight. We start Ben on the demo disk as soon as school is over and we get the computer set up. Then we break for two weeks, subscribe to the online account, and start the formal program."

John nodded as he ate a forkful of his mashed potatoes.

"We take our vacation to see your folks in Colorado during his two-week break from playing the demo Fast ForWord. Right?"

"Right."

"We come home and start the actual program with him."

"That's my understanding."

"And you'll take care of all the computer stuff," I repeated.

"Yes."

I twiddled my fork in my food, which was now almost cold. "She also said we needed to set up a behavior modification or reward system for him," I said as much to myself as to John. "I'll have to go and get some small toys. Peter will want them, too, you know."

John grinned. "More than likely."

"Okay." I exhaled. "Can we do this?"

"Sure. You're the smartest person I know."

I rolled my eyes. "Doesn't this make you nervous as hell?"

"No." And he kept on eating.

"Why did it take so long to know, John?" I repeated the question, now in a rhetorical, exhausted way.

His hands froze, and his eyes focused on me as if I was accusing him of not adequately diagnosing our son.

I touched his hand to reassure him. "I mean, if we've never heard of auditory processing disorder, think of how many other people haven't. It explains so much of what we've seen in Ben. The big riddle is finally solved." I glanced at Ben and lowered my voice. "He's bright, but he can't talk. Give him an instruction and you're out of luck, but add a visual cue and you're successful." I murmured, "He couldn't understand us."

We ate in silence the rest of the time. Ben's fatigue was obvious. He consumed his food quickly and quietly. His chubby fingers reached for his glass of milk.

"Ben, I love you. It's going to be okay now. We're going to do some things that might help you." I smiled at him, wishing I could hold him in my arms.

"Okay. Tanks," he said before finishing his milk.

Emotions filled me, and I laid my fork down on my empty plate. I didn't remember eating any of it. The feelings melted and beat together inside me. Anger—after years of misdiagnoses and confusion. Relief—that we'd discovered the truth. Sadness—that my child had suffered through the years, that his anxiety had a real and well-founded explanation. That he couldn't have told me himself since he'd never been able to process sounds normally. Grief—because those years were lost to us, and the picture of a child who was fine wasn't true. Overwhelmed—that there was so very much to do and learn.

GLORIA'S FORMAL TESTING REPORT CAME A FEW DAYS LATER. I was alone; both of the boys were at school when I drove down to get the mail. I flipped through the envelopes once back inside the house, and I felt a little dizzy when the clinic letterhead appeared. I threw the other mail aside and tore open the envelope. It was as I'd expected and dreaded. Horrible test scores. A friend and mother of a son who struggled had once told me "your child is more than what's on that piece of paper." Intellectually, I knew that. Emotionally, it was devastating. It seemed as if the years of speech therapy and all the work with Anju had made such marginal differences in Ben's ability to express himself. The hours of driving, all of Ben's hard work, just seemed for nothing.

I started to read the pages in my hand more closely and read them softly out loud to myself. Gloria had done the TAPS-R, or Test of Auditory Perceptual Skills; the CELF-3 or Clinical Evaluation of Language Fundamentals; the SCAN; and an audiological evaluation or hearing tests.

Results of the TAPS-R indicate significant struggle with all auditory perceptual tasks. The Auditory Perceptual Quotient of 56 places Ben's abilities in the extremely low range. Ben was unable to recall digits, unrelated word strings or sentences. . . .

I closed my eyes, and then opened them. I wanted to read it, lay it aside, and be done with it. The results from the CELF-3 were just as bad. Words to describe Ben such as "immature grammar," "telegraphic output," and "stereotypic language" cut into me. Gloria summarized her findings:

Results indicate a pervasive communication disorder affecting both receptive and expressive domains. Language processing skills are reduced sec-

ondary to abnormal auditory perceptive, central auditory processing deficits, and an inability to retrieve known words for commenting and describing. Expressive language is functional for social purposes in familiar situations and with familiar listeners.

My fingers had left depressions on the page, but I mentally thanked Gloria for her last statement. Ben's audiological workup included an otoscopic inspection, pure tone audiometry, and speech discrimination scores under quiet. All the tests revealed normal external structures and bilateral hearing.

The last page recommended further assessment of Ben's intellectual abilities and attentional abilities at another clinic. John and I had discussed this and knew the clinic Gloria was recommending. It was a fine group of clinicians, but we felt nobody knew Ben as well as we did and only God knew what his potential was. Our suspicions of the system were at an all-time high, and we weren't going to let anyone tell us what our six-year-old son's prognosis was, based on a one-second snapshot when we had a video camera running twenty-four hours a day—not when we were finally understanding the riddle.

I stood up and decided I needed more information. I logged onto AOL and briefly checked my e-mail messages. Rosa wanted to know how the evaluation went. I felt I finally had something hopeful to share with her. My sisters had checked in, also concerned. After sending some brief responses, I went to web search and typed "Central Auditory Processing Disorder." A single page of websites appeared. I hit the first one—a link with Learning Disabilities online and waited.

My eyes raced along the screen, soaking up the descriptions, symptoms, and signs of the disorder. The information matched Ben's presentation and behaviors exactly. At least part of it did. It seemed that APD was a very heterogeneous disorder, as Gloria had said, with different kids displaying different difficulties. Some kids had a history of ear infections and some didn't. Some had difficulties with speech while others didn't. But the bottom line for each of the children was distortion in the way they processed sounds. A routine hearing test wouldn't pick it up. A Canadian website described the difficulty some academic communities were having in accepting APD as a diagnosis.

Advances in understanding and strategies to help children with auditory processing disorder had happened within the past ten years. Controversy in framing the disorder, models subscribed to, and etiology—why these kids had it—surrounded the disorder. Was APD related to chronic ear infections? Or was it due to a familial link? Perinatal trauma? More controversial opinions were thrown into the discussions on parent listservs regarding the causes of APD: maternal hypothyroidism, and immune and vitamin deficiencies were just a few mentioned by parents seeking to make sense of the disorder.

The more I read, the more inexact the answers and theories seemed to be. Unfortunately, aside from a few academic discussions, which were too expensive and jargon-filled for the layperson, there were no books to help parents. Only the Internet, with its various websites, provided information. But the Internet was a place where anything by anyone could be posted, a new frontier where the quacks and the scholars alike had equal access. I saw a sad gap between what was available and the real world of parents struggling desperately to help their children.

It struck me now how easily a child like Ben, who had a severe problem, could be mistaken for being mentally handicapped, autistic, or having attention problems. Yet the root of this difficulty diverged greatly from the others. This was an input problem, not an output problem, nor one of intellect, nor one of a social, psychological, or emotional nature.

I shifted my chair a bit and hit another site. A mother of a young girl who had APD had started this one. There was a link to a simulation of APD, an audio demonstration. I hit go, and a picture of a wolf came into view with sentences of words I couldn't read. The title at the top said, "Ladle Rat Rotten Hut." A woman's voice came through the speakers. Gibberish, yet with inflections and pauses between sentences. The words were printed in gibberish as well, nonsensical words without meaning.

As I listened to the story of "Little Red Riding Hood," I brushed the tears aside, slapping my cheeks to be rid of them, and realized that this was how Ben had been hearing his whole life.

CHAPTER TEN

I Can Hear That

IT WAS THE CHILDREN'S PROGRAM NIGHT, MARKING THE END of the school year. Ben had completed his kindergarten year and would be advancing to first grade. Miss Mary had cleared it with Miss Rice, the first-grade teacher, assuring her he demonstrated the necessary skills. Peter had finished his first year of preschool and was due to have his fourth birthday in a few months.

Tonight, both Peter and Ben would be singing with their preschool classes. Although the weather was totally different, the evening reminded me of the December night a year and a half ago, when Ben had been led around the stage at the Christmas pageant. I sighed and looked behind to see the boys, sitting with their white T-shirts on, specially decorated by the kids for tonight's show. They had their names on them and the outline of an animal. Peter's had a kangaroo and Ben's had a fish.

"You think Ben will be okay?" I asked John.

He looked in the rearview mirror at Ben. "I think so."

"You okay, Ben?" I asked.

He seemed extra quiet. "What I do?"

"You just sing the songs you've been practicing. You'll be standing with your friends and Miss Mary will be right there."

Peter chimed in, "It'll be fun. We get to stand up on the big stage."

"That's right. It will be fun, Pete."

Ben blinked and swallowed.

"You'll both do great." I shot John a glance, trying to let him know that we needed to make sure Ben was okay.

The auditorium was beyond hot. It was ovenlike and filled with children ranging in age from two to twelve. Children, teachers, and parents talking, screaming, and crying rolled into a wave of noise. The four of us were directed to the back entrance of the auditorium to drop the kids off. Ben saw Miss Mary and smiled. Then Frank, his friend, greeted him and they quickly put their arms over one another's shoulders so that I could snap their picture.

I left Ben, ecstatic that when he saw familiar faces, he was able to relax, and went in search of Peter's class and teacher. On the other side of the large, crowded, baking room, was Mrs. Minett, another gifted teacher at the school. A woman in her mid-fifties, she had elegance about her, a petite frame, and a wonderful amount of energy in keeping up with her preschoolers. She looked fresh despite the heat and opened her arms to Peter. He saw some playmates, and we shouted a good-bye to him. John and I went around the building to secure our seats in the almost filled theater.

I chatted with John about his job. He'd taken a small pay cut, but the position matched John's strengths in many ways—his experiences with medically unstable psychiatric patients, his work with adults over the recent years, and his ability to handle the competing needs of the two organizations diplomatically. Although it'd been painful at times, John had grown as a professional. And he definitely felt needed. It was such a demanding position that the other doctors at the clinic hadn't wanted it.

"I'm so glad, John." I squeezed his arm, then noticed John's face had tilted forward to address someone in the aisle. It was Mrs. Minett.

Her voice was low as she bent over to speak with us. "Peter is having some difficulty. He's pretty upset."

"Should I come for him?" I grabbed the handle of my purse.

"Well, not right now. I think I have him calmed down enough." She waved her hands slightly. "But you may want to watch the stage and see if he's okay."

John said, "What if he's not?"

"See that stairway over there?" She motioned toward a side set of steps. "Watch for my signal and if he gets too upset, come up and get him off the stage."

I nodded. Clearly, this had happened to other kids. "Is he crying?"

"Yes. But I think he'll be all right. He just needs to get used to the bigness of it all."

She waved good-bye hurriedly, indicating her place was with the kids.

I shifted uncomfortably in my seat. Poor Pete. He was always so sure of himself, but underneath, he was just a little boy. The guilt from my benign neglect filled me once again. I wanted to go get my blond-haired boy, the one with the slightly buck teeth from sucking on his pacifier. I wanted to hold him and tell him from now on, I'd be a better mother to him. I scanned the auditorium and stage and tried to picture it from the perspective of my younger son.

I blurted out, "What are we going to do?"

"Let's see how he does." John, too, had taken up a constant stare at the stage.

"Look, why don't you position yourself down there in case he's upset?"

Before I was finished, John had stood up. "See you later." I watched him take a spot beneath the brightly lit stage. The lights dimmed just as John took his position.

The program began with the two-year-olds, who were barely able to sing every other word, but got high marks in being adorable. Peter's class was next. I straightened my back and neck, craning to see Pete. He was at the side, just a few feet from the stairs. Mrs. Minett crouched low, comforting him from behind. His nose was red and he looked totally petrified. His mouth hung open, his eyes were wide and glazed over. No movement at all. Peter spotted John, and he immediately held his arms out to his dad. John moved quickly up the stairs, scooped him off the edge of the stage, and brought him to my side.

Peter was trying not to cry, and I put him on my lap where he curled against me. "My boy. It's okay. Mama's here."

"It was scary." He started to cry in full force. "Why does there have to be those bright lights?"

I smoothed his hair away from his sweaty forehead and kept kissing his face, soothing him with soft words.

Ben did fine. He sang his songs with his class, his body loose, his arms and hands moving to the motions he'd been taught. Then when the preschool classes had finished, we found Ben seated with his classmates, and all of us went home.

JOHN AND I PURCHASED A NEW COMPUTER THAT MATCHED the Fast ForWord specifications that Gloria had given us. I watched John take the various pieces of hardware and cables out of the boxes. Without a glance at the instructions, his fingers found each portal and hookup. I marveled at how he knew what went where and the ease with which he did it.

Two good-quality headphones were also necessary for playing the computer program: one set for Ben to wear and one set for the monitor—in this case, John or me. We signed up with a full-service Internet provider that would allow us to download Ben's data after each day of play. The summer months had just begun. And we started the demo.

I'd assigned John the task of working with Ben. John agreed that while he played the Fast ForWord demo with Ben, I'd watch Pete. I softly stepped downstairs on the first night to see how it was going. Gloria had said to play for about a half hour.

I stood behind John and Ben, trying not to disturb them.

Each of them wore his headphones, and Ben's little head leaned toward the computer screen as the exercises unfolded. I could hear the sound as it escaped from their headphones and listened at the computer's stretched-out voice that seemed to open up a new auditory world to Ben. John noticed me, turned, and gave thumbs up.

A few minutes later, they finished the games for the day, and Ben headed upstairs for a snack.

"How's he doing?" I said.

John paused and took off his headphones. "Great. He seems to like to do it. Some games are easier than others for him, but I have trouble with the prompts sometimes."

I rolled my eyes. "The branch doesn't fall far from the tree, does it?" And gave him a kiss on the cheek.

John chuckled and shut down the computer.

"Do you think this will help him?" I crossed my arms and thought of the thousands of dollars invested. The time involved. The commitment. The responsibility of doing it at home. What if it didn't work?

John carefully put the headphones beside the computer. "I think so. We can only try. We can only give it our best shot."

DEMO PLAY CONTINUED FOR THE NEXT TWO WEEKS, PROVIDing each of the Fast ForWord games for an abbreviated time period: about five minutes of play instead of twenty. The booklet that came with the CD disk from Scientific Learning Corporation described the seven games, five of which were played daily on a rotating basis.

The first was Circus Sequence or CS. In this game, Ben saw various circus animals position themselves at the top of the screen. He heard two sounds—one high and one low—in different sequences. He needed to replicate the order of the sounds by clicking on the orange triangle and pink square. The speed of the stimuli was amazing. It struck me that no human could provide such repetitive and rapid input.

The second game was called Old Macdonald's Flying Farm or OMDFF. Ben would see a flying object from a farm—a chick in a basket, for example—slowly coming down across the screen. He had to catch the flying animal and hold the mouse button down until he detected the delicate change in sound. The voice might say, "Gi, Gi, Gi, Gi, Gi, Gi, Gi, Ki." If Ben didn't respond when it changed from Gi to Ki, the figure would fly off into the sky.

The third game was called Phoneme Identification or PI. The challenge to this game was to identify an individual phoneme over a competing one. An identified phoneme would be chosen for Ben, such as "ba." Then two animal characters would appear in the screen facing each other and in quick succession say similar phonemes, such as "ba" and "da." As soon as Ben hit the target phoneme character, he would earn his points and the game would continue.

The fourth game was Phonic Words or PW. This challenged Ben to distinguish words that differed only by an initial consonant (such as "tack" or "pack") or a final consonant (such as "pat" and "pack"). Again a target word was identified for Ben, such as "rake," with a distracter such as "lake." This was one of the easiest games for Ben.

The fifth game was called Phonic Match or PM, and it reminded me of an old game show. Every time Ben clicked on a tile, he'd hear a sound or word. He had to find the other tile with the matching sound or word, using as few clicks of the mouse as possible. The game started with four tiles, but could progress to sixteen tiles.

Block Commander or BC was the name of the sixth game. A three-dimensional checkerboard, with a cat peering over the top, had different colored squares and circles lined up in parallel horizontal rows. Ben was given a command to manipulate the shapes, such as "Touch the small blue square" and "Put the green square behind the white circle."

The last game was called Language Comprehension Builder or LCB. I recognized this as the game Ben had played in Gloria's office. A sentence was read to Ben and the screen split into two to four pictures—one picture depicted what the sentence said. Ben heard: "The boy is being pushed by the girl." He saw four pictures, one of a boy being pushed in a wagon by a clown, one of a clown being pushed by a girl, one of a girl being pushed by a boy, and the correct one.

After coming home from a long day at work, John would faithfully retreat into the basement with Ben and set up the demo games. We were already getting a clear sense of which games were the most difficult for him: Circus Sequence, Phoneme Identification, Block Commander, and Language Comprehension Builder. He seemed to lack the skills to identify distinct phonemes and high/low tones, and to understand sentences as they became increasingly more complex.

WE WERE SCHEDULED TO LEAVE FOR COLORADO IN THE UP-coming days, and I had mixed feelings. The last time I'd gone, I'd ended up in the hospital and cradled a wound with every bounce back during the twenty-one-hour drive home. Still, the boys needed to know their grandparents. I was in the kitchen looking over my to-do list and heard Ben saying something to himself, and then call out, "Mom."

I got up from the table and went to where he stood by the aquarium. He was still drawn to water and the living creatures in it. He loved watching the small minnows we'd scooped up from our lake swim about. He seemed transfixed as he stared into the corner where bubbles streamed up to the top of the water from the filter.

"Ben?"

He turned away from the soft sound and looked at me. "I can hear that." He pointed to the bubbles.

"What?" I whispered.

He pointed one of his little fingers to the aquarium. "I can hear that."

"And you couldn't hear it before?" My voice was gentle, my mind wanting to understand and savor this victory with him.

His brown eyes went from the bubbles to my face. "No." He broke out into a smile, keeping his finger pointed.

I reached over and hugged him, laughing and crying at the same time. "Ben, that's wonderful." I broke away. "You can hear it now?" I repeated.

He nodded, smiled and pressed his fingers against the glass, watching the minnows dance gracefully and show us flashes of silver as the sunlight hit their bodies. And yet I knew he had been able to "hear" sounds before, sometimes too acutely. This program seemed to bring his ability to process aural sounds in a new way. I rejoiced with my son. Now he could perceive the beauty in the world around him, instead of hearing just noise.

OTHER THAN HAVING OUR CAR BREAK DOWN THREE TIMES— once on the way to Colorado and twice coming home—and al- most being stranded in a stretch of godforsaken flatlands, we had a nice visit. Prior to leaving, John and I had decided to tell Peter we'd forgotten to pack his pacifier, hoping he would have no choice but to go "cold-turkey." All our previous attempts had failed, and we were desperate to get our almost four-year-old off it. Peter, being the extremely bright kid he was, had looked at us after about three hours of pacifier withdrawal and said, "You guys are trying to trick me."

John and I had broken down, confessing our ruse and had set up a reward system if he would kick the pacifier habit. It had worked, and we'd come back from Colorado pacifier free. These vacations always left me eternally grateful for my home, the short drive to the mailbox, and the thick Midwest air. I was even glad to see the dogs and my old, mean cat.

I'd planned a busy summer for Ben and included Pete as much as I could. Bridget and I had planned for play dates with her boys and mine at a large nearby state park pool. I thought that swim- ming, one of the skills Ben had a natural talent in, would be help- ful to his sensory integration issues. It would also provide an outlet for both his and Peter's energy. Swimming seemed to give

Ben focus and the ability to attend more. It relaxed him. The body movements in the water helped to give him mental and physical balance.

John and I signed the kids up for a six-week summer school session at the Montessori school. In fact, they'd be in the same classroom together with Miss Mary and another great teacher who had worked with Ben in kindergarten.

I'd also made contact with the children's clinic for an OT recheck on Ben's fine motor skills. I knew first grade included more writing and other tasks requiring hand strength and coordination. It was great to see everyone, especially Anju, whom we greeted with a hug, and Elizabeth, who assessed him and concluded the following:

Generally improved control was observed with small muscle motor/manipulative tasks. Ben is able to complete manipulative tasks at a more functional speed. However, rate of execution could increase. Ben is a delightful young man with the diagnosis of auditory processing difficulty. He is demonstrating emerging self-confidence with his fine motor skills and self-awareness. Fine motor skills are mildly to moderately delayed.

Two rechecks were scheduled. Elizabeth supplied me with a folder containing a home-based program that she felt could be incorporated into his summer school curriculum. There were exercises for copying and cutting. I gave it to Mary on his next day at school.

Gloria officially registered us with Scientific Learning Corporation, the company that produced and distributed Fast ForWord. She gave us a client number, a password, and her provider number that were necessary to access the system and download the data. Although John monitored Ben during the demo games, that arrangement wasn't going to work when Ben was expected to play 100 minutes per day, five days out of seven. So I took over.

We planned Ben's play days as Wednesday through Sunday with Monday and Tuesday off. He attended summer school Monday through Thursday, so the only days when school and Fast ForWord overlapped were Wednesday and Thursday.

I'd arranged for Joanne's daughter to sit during the first couple of weeks to help with Peter. She was like a member of the family, and she'd intermittently watched Ben since we moved to the area when he was six months old.

The first official day of Fast ForWord arrived. John had oriented me on the downloading procedure; the sitter was upstairs watching Peter; Ben finished his lunch and was ready to play. I loaded the CD, and the games began. The booklet showed me the rotation of the seven games, with five being played each day. I was all set. Now it was up to Ben.

Circus Sequence began and Ben clicked away, with excellent attention to the game. Each game lasted twenty minutes, much longer than the span he was used to.

"Beep/Beep." A high/low combination. Ben clicked the triangle and the square, earning two points on the ticker at the top of the screen.

"That's great!" I said.

Ben continued, starting out strong. But as his fatigue increased, he started to miss.

"Slow down, honey. You're going too fast."

Ben didn't look away from the screen. The sounds continued just as soon as he clicked the mouse. Ben's eyes darted away from the triangle and square to see how many points he'd earned, which he did for the remaining four games of the day.

By the end of the first day's play, I felt exhilarated and fatigued. "Thank you, Ben, for working so hard," I shouted to him as he was already halfway up the stairs. But he stopped and came back to watch and listen to the clapping and whistling noise that accompanied the sound and image of coins being stacked into towers. As it finished, we were told how many tokens he'd earned for the day.

"You did great, Ben!" He gave me a grin and ran upstairs to see Peter.

I got online and downloaded his first day's data without any problem. I had known it was going to be a challenge, but I glanced at my watch and realized it was time to make dinner.

* * *

THE SECOND DAY CAME TOO SOON FOR BEN, WHO THOUGHT it was a one-day thing and that he could choose to play or not. The third day and fourth day were even harder. He was genuinely worn out by the fifth day.

By the end of the second week, I had a revolt on my hands.

"Ben, Gloria said we *have* to play. The schedule says so." I held up the calendar that came with the data report. It marked each day that the program was played. "And I'll give you a toy."

"Big one." It wasn't a question, it was a demand.

"Okay." I eyed him, thinking what was in my toy stash. "Only if you really try and don't give me a hard time."

He eyed me, sizing up my resolve. "I do it." His words carried a message that he was doing this for me and in a way, he was.

I rubbed his back after he sat down. He promptly plunked down his headphones over his curly hair and over his ears. "Let's just do it and get it over with. Then we get two days off."

He turned. "Two days?"

"Yep."

"You sit here whole time?"

"Whole time."

I loaded the disk, and we settled into the games. Once the games began, he attended well. Although I could see the games made him nervous at times, especially when he chose the wrong answer, he never quit trying. The machine just kept going and expected Ben to do the same.

GLORIA'S CLINIC HAD GIVEN US PROGRESS NOTE SHEETS TO monitor the time spent on the games, Ben's level of frustration, and the level of assistance needed. I also charted comments about what seemed to help Ben the most. On day ten, I noted: "PM— new sound grid. CS—misses low/high sequence the most. BC is hard for Ben. I worked the mouse. But he's getting better at repeating and understanding the commands."

Gloria e-mailed me daily with comments and an attachment of Ben's data analysis, trials attempted, and a bar graph that showed his performance for the day, based upon percent of the game completed. At times, I thought he'd done better than the data analysis reflected. Gloria would write encouraging e-mail notes:

Don't get discouraged. Ben's data looks very good for this early in the program. On BC, if you can get him to put the mouse pointer on the spot as soon as he hears the first direction—such as "put the white circle"— and then listen for the next piece—such as "next to the blue square"—he will probably do better. This game is going to take time. Hang in there. Gloria.

The data fascinated me. I held Week Three's summary in my hands and flipped through the pages. For OMDFF, Ben had rocketed to 94% completion. He'd had 179 trials of "gi–ki," 220 trials of "chu–shu," 158 trials of "si–sti," 115 trials of "ge–ke," and 158 trials of "do–to." This program, that seemed to be changing my son's brain functioning, was delivering stimuli via technology in a manner that a human being was simply incapable of doing. The machine did it without pauses, without hesitation. It didn't have to look at its notes or find its place, or decide if Ben's answer was correct. It adapted the stimuli to his ability. All this was immediate and continuous.

The other games displayed similar specifics, but with different completion percentages: BC was at 27%; CS was at 9% and had become much more difficult for Ben; PM was at 33%; PW was at 17%; PI was at 17% and had also become challenging for him as it adapted to his performance. LCB was at 16%. Still, Gloria was encouraged by his progress, and I started to see small, but noticeable changes in Ben that were verified by Jamie, his tutor. I shared these impressions with Gloria:

It dawned on me yesterday while I was talking to Ben's tutor that he doesn't ask "huh?" anymore. My rate of having to repeat messages to him has decreased, I'd say, by about 80%. It's wonderful. For both of us. His tutor saw more of the child coming out in Ben—his personality, his wit and humor. She also says his ability to say a word phonetically is drasti-

cally improved. I'm glad he has a couple of days off. He was pretty pooped by the end of Day Five. If there's anything I should do differently, let me know. Or any suggestions. He needs to slow down during CS. He's in too much of a hurry. Thanks so much again. Karen.

THE SUMMER PROGRESSED, AS DID OUR FAMILY LIFE, AROUND Fast ForWord. We didn't leave town on the weekends because we didn't want to interrupt Ben's schedule. We stopped going to church, as Sunday mornings were his time to play. I was completely obsessed with the program. I felt like a general of a one-man army, ordering Ben to do the games on days when neither of us felt like doing them. But we faithfully kept to the schedule.

I clung to the plan for the summer desperately, compulsively, and with a feeling that finally, I was doing something significant for Ben. I tried not to think about the follow-up testing. I trusted what I was seeing and hearing. But the chant inside kept growing stronger: Is it enough? Will he catch up? Is it enough? Will he catch up?

We stuck to the reward system for Ben, and if Peter behaved during the time Ben played, he would also get a reward. I scoured the toy clearance aisles for small items that I thought the boys would like and had managed to keep a decent collection handy. I'd also noticed that when I let Ben swim prior to playing Fast ForWord, his performance was usually better. He focused and didn't get as frustrated.

It wasn't necessary for the sitter to come anymore, and Peter was usually pretty compliant with Ben's time on the computer. I felt, though, as if I were pushing Peter away at times. Ben insisted on me being present every minute. His anxiety when he didn't know something was cushioned by my comments: "It's okay, Ben. Just try again," "You'll get it next time," "Slow down," or "It's just one answer, Ben. The important thing is that you learn why you missed."

But Peter, who just celebrated his fourth birthday, wanted me to spend time with him, too. To work a puzzle or mold Play-Doh.

His inquisitive nature grew hourly with "why" questions that showed amazing thought. His queries stumped me more times than I cared to admit. I tried to include Peter by allowing him to listen with the headphones at times, but distractions made Ben lose focus and miss. It was best if Peter stayed away from the computer.

By Week Six, Ben's fatigue started to become more pronounced, as did his lower tolerance for frustration. It took more prompting for him to get started. The boys had finished summer school, so we had the whole day free of outside activities. Less structure in the morning wasn't necessarily a good thing.

"Come on, Ben. Let's get started."

"Again and again and again." The whine in his voice rose as he bent his head back. He'd collapsed on the sofa, a cartoon capturing his attention.

"Ben, I told you after your last show, it was time. It's raining today so you can't swim. Let's just get it over with." I walked away, hoping he'd follow. Peter was sitting at the kitchen table, playing with a new Lego building block creation of his. "Peter, Mommy is going downstairs. If you have to go to the bathroom, just do like Daddy showed you, okay? If you have trouble, call me."

Peter and I had decided it was time for him to be potty-trained. His big gray-blue eyes blinked, and I wished I had eyelashes as long as Peter's. "Okay, Mommy. I like big boy pants." He grinned.

"Let's go one more time before I start the computer with Ben."

After taking Peter for his few drops of relief in the toilet, I yelled for my other son. "Come on, Ben. You'll get a toy after you play." I waited, aware of my blatant bribery, and felt a millisecond of guilt. If it got the job done, at this point, who cared?

I saw him saunter toward me, sullen and with a closed mouth. I rubbed his arm. "Look, I know it's hard on some days. Let's just get started."

"I get toy?" he said, stopping until he got an answer.

"Yes. Like always." Then I added, "I don't think we play the Cat Game today." He absolutely hated this game.

He looked up sharply. "No Cat Game?" He smiled and started down the steps.

We got the games up and running. Both Ben and I groaned when the Cat Game or Block Commander did appear. I'd read the schedule wrong and apologized to Ben. His eyes scolded me.

"Well, we have to do it, honey. Lean forward toward the screen." I stood up and scooted his chair closer to the table—not easy, with his seated husky body. "Sit up straight. That's it."

We were halfway through. "That's the way, Ben. Put the mouse on the first object you hear and then listen and repeat what they say."

His little head seemed so much bigger with the headphones on. I'd tilted mine to the side so I could also listen for Peter.

"Good, Ben. You got—"

"Mommy!" It was Peter, yelling from upstairs. "I peed my big boy pants!"

"Damn," I muttered. "Ben, I gotta go help your brother."

"No! Don't leave."

"I'll be right back."

I ran up the stairs and almost bumped into Pete's crying face. "It just came all of a sudden."

"It's okay, honey. You're doing good. You're just getting used to this."

His face brightened a bit. "Yeah."

"Those pull-on diaper thingies felt bulky, and these are a lot thinner. You'll get the hang of it. We just have to make sure we try to go potty all the time."

"Okay, Mommy." After I helped Peter change, I threw the growing pile of clothes into the laundry room and went back to help Ben. I'd done the right thing, leaving Ben alone. He'd done all right in my absence, and it gave me satisfaction to have been able to put Peter's needs first.

*　*　*

BY THE END OF WEEK SIX, BEN'S DATA LOOKED GOOD. HE
had completed OMDFF and PW. Three games—PM, LCB, and
BC—were all in the 70% completed range. But by far the two
most challenging games were Circus Sequence (56%) and
Phoneme Identification (52%). All the games had adapted to
Ben's progress. The signals came more frequently. The weekly
analysis provided specific information on what Ben did each day
and what were the most difficult tasks. For example, on PI, distinguishing among three phonemes pairs "bi–di," "be–de," and
"aba–ada" was extremely frustrating for Ben. Sometimes, I had a
hard time telling the difference.

Overall, however, Gloria was very pleased. Regardless of what
Ben's scores might have said, I continued to see real effects in his
daily life. I wrote to Gloria:

*Last night, Ben's "best buddy," Frank, called him on the telephone—
they haven't seen each other since the beginning of June. Ben was able to
hear his friend and made some decent conversation with him. For example, he talked about a Batman movie he'd seen, about Bible school's party
with pizza, and other topics appropriate for a six-year-old boy. While it
wasn't the best grammar or sentence structure I've ever heard, he was able
to hear his friend speak and contribute to the dialogue. Ben's really
missed this little boy. It was a real milestone for him. Thanks, Karen.*

Yet as much as I celebrated these new accomplishments, I
couldn't help but feel the glaring lags between Ben and his peers.
I'd heard almost miraculous stories about the program, and while
seeing great gains already, I wondered if a miracle was in our future. The summer was luxurious. No academics to worry about.
No driving to and fro. I knew the fall was coming, and I tried not
to spoil the days by being negative, but inside I felt like Judgment Day was coming all too soon.

THE FOLLOWING SUNDAY, MOTIVATED BY JOHN'S PAY CUT, I
picked up the *Indianapolis Star* and scanned the classified ads.
One caught my attention immediately. It was an ad for medical

writers placed by the premier pharmaceutical company in Indianapolis. I had always wanted to work for this company, but wasn't sure in what capacity. I located the company's website and read the job description for medical writer. A perfect fit. It would combine my background in social sciences research and writing skills.

John and I discussed it. Despite my protests that it would be difficult for me to commute an hour and fifteen minutes each way and still keep everything going at home, he encouraged me to find out more information because he knew I wanted to. I called the number and was able to set up an interview. The recruiter in charge of hiring medical writers told me to expect a writing test in the mail and to send it back before the interview.

It arrived a few days later, in the form of a scientific article on the efficacy of a certain drug. I needed to write a synopsis, making sure it contained certain points. The article described a typical study—with hypotheses, data collection, data analysis, weaknesses of the study noted, and conclusions. I woke up early the next morning—since morning was when I did my best work—and started to write the summary.

Still in my robe, I curled up on the living room sofa and positioned my coffee, pen, and paper just so. I began to read about the study design, how the subjects were selected, how the data was analyzed, and how statistical significance was determined. It was intoxicating. Mental muscles long dormant and atrophied began flexing and moving stiffly, but surely. I felt a rush as I sighed in relief that I not only understood what was being discussed but I could also see the faults in design and conclusions.

There was sound from upstairs. I froze and my pen stopped on the page. My ears detected footsteps from Peter's bedroom. I was almost done, but needed a few more minutes to myself. But there was Peter, blond hair sticking up on one side and mashed on the other, rubbing his eyes, looking at me and saying, "What's for breakfast, Mommy?"

* * *

THE DAY OF THE INTERVIEW CAME, A STEAMY, UNCOMFORTABLE day that made me think whoever invented pantyhose never had to wear them on a hot, humid Indiana day. With the car's air conditioning kept at high, I arrived slightly wrinkled, but not too damp.

In the middle of the front circular drive, six feet of vertical water gushed from a fountain. As I felt the cool spray on my arms, I longed to jump in. The corporate center's doors were elegantly curved in frosted glass, reflecting the fluidity in the total architectural design. I walked into the air-conditioned room and stood in wonder. High ceilings and plush carpet intermingled with shiny floor tiles, women wearing New York's finest fashions, their makeup bold, but becoming, and people walking briskly about behind the roped-off desk that I approached.

Two guards stood stiffly, watching by the two ports of entry behind the desk. I was issued a temporary nametag, which popped out of a computer within seconds. I was instructed to have a seat at the far end of the room until my contact person came to escort me into the building. I placed my briefcase on the floor and just took it all in. I heard the name of the Indianapolis school superintendent being called. I recognized the woman who stood up from her appearances on the six o'clock news.

Then a man, wearing a casual pair of khaki pants and a shirt with no tie, came toward me and offered his hand. "Hi. Karen?"

"Yes. Mr. Joiner?"

He nodded. "Brad, please." He explained that the interview would take place in an adjoining building. We walked down a hallway, rode an elevator, went down a few steps, and walked around cubicles and orange office walls. He was a young pup, but seemed nice with his boyish dark hair and open smile. Not what I'd expected.

His office was a walled-off cubicle with a computer and a few papers lying on the horseshoe-shaped counter. He explained that we'd have a bit of a wait, and I'd be interviewed by the two members of the writing team and then by the manager in charge. We chatted about an antidepressant drug the company was famous for, and I gave my opinion on the impact it had had not only on the view of depression in society, but on how managed care had used it in some ways as an excuse to bypass therapy.

His phone rang, and we were off to meet the writers. I sat down in an even smaller area, more like a booth crammed with a table, an easel with erasable markers, and six chairs. Each member of the team came individually to interview me. There was an MBA in a starched white shirt with gold cuff links who had no experience with medical writing, but was newly hired himself and getting the hang of it. A senior member of the team with a background in nursing, like me, who asked some tough questions about my vita and my short tenure on most of my previous jobs. I explained that I'd left many of the positions to pursue further educational opportunities and, more recently, due to marriage.

The manager was the sister of a woman I'd attended high school with. I shifted uneasily in my seat, embarrassed by the weight I'd gained and my lack of professional activity over the past seven years. She showed me an example of a report the team had compiled. "Pretty dry stuff, isn't it? Are you sure after writing fiction that this would satisfy you?"

I glanced through the pages—a fat, turbo-charged scientific treatise on a drug that had been thoroughly investigated over many clinical trials by many different individuals. "Well, I'm familiar with this type of work. I wouldn't think there'd be room for suspense or mystery." We chuckled. "But yeah. This is fine by me."

We talked for a little while longer, and when the interview was concluded, we left the booth and found Brad waiting nearby. He told me they'd be in touch within the next few days, as they were interviewing two other applicants. I left feeling pumped up. The interview had gone well. And I was uneasy. This would be a great job, but a nagging voice kept asking just how I was going to be able to make it work.

* * *

TRUE TO HIS WORD, BRAD CALLED A COUPLE OF DAYS LATER, offering me a full-time position. He'd had a chance to talk with the other members of the team, and they felt I'd work out well. My writing test looked good, and he had no doubt I'd make a great medical writer. He then offered me a salary that was more money than I'd ever made in my life.

"Would you consider part-time?" I asked tentatively.

"No, I'm afraid all our writers are full-time. They take on more of a coordinator's job and make sure the physician, statistician, and other people who make up the clinical trial team are on-board with their parts."

"What about job sharing?" A member of my writers group and an editor of an educational press had agreed to job share with me.

"An employee who job shares has to have worked with the company for a time before we can allow that type of arrangement."

"Do you have flex-time hours?"

"Yes." He seemed relieved that there was something he could offer. "Many of our writers work six A.M. to three or so in the afternoon. Of course if there's a deadline, that has to be taken into consideration. And there are core hours in the afternoon that we require all employees to be present for so that we can schedule meetings."

"Can I get back with you? I need to talk it over with my husband."

"I'll need to know soon."

"I'll call you tomorrow."

LATER THAT EVENING, JOHN AND I DISCUSSED THE VARIOUS scenarios. Ben and Peter were playing in the living room. John looked spent. He was seeing a lot of suffering and felt frustrated that he couldn't offer more, particularly for substance abuse. Services had dwindled to a trickle.

I started to clear the supper dishes. "Okay, so if I went in early, say around six o'clock, then you'd have to get the kids to school, and then I could try to pick them up." I added, more to myself, than to John, "I'd have to get up around four in the morning."

John rinsed out the coffee pot, watching the dark liquid go down the drain. "Yes."

"What if I have a deadline to meet and have to stay, and I can't pick them up?"

"I'll do it." He met my eyes, and I knew he wanted this for me.

"What if there's an emergency at the hospital, and you're detained? It happens all the time. What about snow days? Which one of us would call in? What about if one of the kids was sick? Which one of us would miss work? What about Ben?"

"He's doing good." He seemed surprised.

"He's not there yet. He's not nearly there."

"But he's come a long way."

"Definitely. But we're not done with the first program, and Gloria has mentioned a new follow-up program that's just as intensive."

"If you want this, we'll work it out."

"That's easy to say. What you mean is 'I'd work it out.'"

"No, we'd work it out." He sounded hurt.

"Look, it's not your fault. What would you do if the ER doctor calls you at four and says there's some poor soul who's in the middle of a psychotic episode and needs to be worked up—and I have to stay due to some deadline?"

John was silent. As he loaded the dishwasher, I wiped the table off.

The next day, I called Brad back and turned down the job.

I knew Ben's preschool years were over and first grade represented the first official year of school and academic standards. Ludicrous in a way, to be so apprehensive about my son's first grade. Yet, I dreaded it in many ways. Really, there was no real choice about the job. I still had my writing, although no takers on the medical thrillers I was penning. I'd had another short story accepted in a mystery magazine, and I'd proofed the galley sheets—the final step before publication. Then, the publisher had decided to suspend publication to "take time to smell the roses." I'd gotten two ugly T-shirts as a consolation prize.

But my writing represented more than getting published now. It was part of who I was. Many members of my writers' group had turned into true friends. I'd taken a couple of fiction writing classes over the past few months at an arts center in a nearby town. The classes were offered on Saturdays when John was usually off. I'd learned even more about the rules of the craft and when to break them. And John's faith in me created a new bond between us. He never complained when I wanted time to write, watching the boys while I tried to finish another chapter or revise a new short story.

And Rosa and I drifted further apart. Whereas before, I was obsessed with Ben's delays and what was causing them, now I was obsessed with Ben's progress and whether or not it would be enough. E-mail had replaced almost all our telephone calls since it was cheaper and more convenient. Yet it had taken something critical from Rosa and me. Personal contact.

I couldn't get out of the boat yet. Or even take one foot out for fear of capsizing. The water's color was changing slightly to more lavender than purple, and if I sat up very straight and strong in the boat, I could make out the faintest sign of a flat piece of shoreline. Peter had joined Ben and me. I had to make sure he was safe as well. He hadn't chosen to be in this water, and I owed him my best.

But night after night, I'd find myself staring at my briefcase before falling asleep. Eventually, it was buried under some clothes that needed mending. Even then, I never forgot it was there.

CHAPTER ELEVEN

A Child's Labor

WE CONTINUED FAST FORWORD FOR THREE MORE WEEKS, with more resistance from Ben. He was tired, and I didn't blame him. He just wanted some downtime when he didn't have to "go to work." I felt the same way, but the pace wasn't going to let up. Ben's final day of Fast ForWord play was a mere two days before the school year began. Again I wondered if it was enough. Had he caught up enough?

Gloria sent me the Nine Week Completion Report for Ben, a detailed report that listed his completion rate for each game and the level of processed sound he was able to negotiate. Ben had met the guidelines for successful discharge from the program: He'd completed five of the seven games with a score of 90% or higher. The remaining two games, Block Commander (75%) and Phoneme Identification (85%), still had respectable ending scores.

Other areas had shown progress as well. Elizabeth had performed a final OT recheck, and I e-mailed Gloria with the good news:

I showed Elizabeth Ben's work from summer school and papers he'd done with his tutor. Elizabeth was pleased and also noted a marked improvement in his concentration and a decrease in his distractibility. She told me that I could bring him back based on the "family initiative." In other words, it's up to John and me. Isn't that great? Karen.

I was proud of my sons. Ben had worked really hard and had learned discipline and shown tenacity. He gave it his all every time he played. Peter, too, had achieved an important milestone: He was now independent in his toileting. Peter was growing from a toddler to a little boy who, although rather impulsive, showed sensitivity to others and had a wonderful sense of humor. After the school program incident, I made sure to check with Peter to see if he was okay, particularly when I thought he was being unusually quiet or didn't feel well. I'd reassure him that I'd take care of him and that there was nothing to worry about.

I looked back over the summer. It had had a magical quality to it, a gift of moving forward with life and of finding some long-awaited answers. In addition to the major strides made with Ben and his auditory processing, I felt a new cohesiveness to the family. By being able to provide the program in the home, I didn't have to take Peter to a sitter or feel guilty about leaving him. Instead of sitting helplessly by as a therapist worked with Ben, I was able to be an active part of his treatment. We were indeed in this together. On Ben's last day of Fast ForWord, I wrote Gloria:

I was so proud of Ben when I got his data—I knew today that something had "clicked" inside of him when he was doing Circus Sequence. He actually did better than I think I would have done. Then this evening, he started to use possessive forms of words and plurals, and smiled and emphasized them when he spoke. His sentence structure is improving steadily. We took a drive and Ben would repeat everything I said to John—even long chains of words! In Phoneme Identification, at the beginning of the program, Ben and I were hearing different phonemes. Today, he and I were hearing the same sounds. It's been quite a wonderful ride. Karen.

THE POST-FAST FORWORD TESTING TOOK PLACE TWO WEEKS later. Again, I sat looking at the woodland creatures in the play area and waited for Gloria to come and get Ben. She greeted us with more familiarity this time, a more relaxed posture. After she and Ben departed, I twitched, shifted in my seat, and made banal small talk with John. I noticed Ben's testing lasted longer, which I found out later was because he was able to do more of the tests.

The receptionist finally invited us back to Gloria's office where we found Ben playing on the floor with some small stuffed animals.

After we sat down, Gloria began her report. "Basically, we've got the receptive component in place now. He's able to process much better than before. His expressive abilities are still severely delayed, however."

"You mentioned another program. A follow-up to Fast For-Word," I said.

"Yes. It's so new that it's not even on the market yet. It's supposed to come out in the next few weeks." She tightened her folded hands in anticipation. "You'll be one of the first families in the country to use it."

I wetted my lips. "What does it do? I mean, is it more of the same?"

Gloria nodded. "Yes, to a certain extent. But it also does some other things. It's meant to build on some of the skills acquired in Fast ForWord or Fast ForWord Language. I will say that Fast For-Word Language to Reading, or Step 4word as it's also called, has more advanced graphics. The child can also choose the order of the games he plays. I've seen them and the games are terrific. I think Ben is an excellent candidate for the program given his success with the first."

"Should we wait a bit? I mean, he's in school now, and he's pretty tired."

Gloria's face became drawn. "He needs it now. I really think you'll see better results if you don't leave too much time between programs. And he's got to navigate school. The more skills we can help him with now, the better off he'll be."

I couldn't argue with her logic as I recalled Ben's kindergarten teacher's gentle warning about him possibly not being able to stay at the Montessori school. So far, first grade was going okay, but when I picked Ben up, Miss Rice's manner made me want to ask if we needed to set up a conference to discuss Ben.

"So is there anything else we should do?"

"Not for right now. But there's another program that I think would suit Ben very well. It's not used too much anymore, since so much speech therapy incorporates play now. But I think it's exactly what Ben needs to build his expressive skills. It's called the *Fokes Sentence Builder,* by Joanne Fokes. It's a program that builds sentences with picture cards. Very structured." Gloria wrinkled her nose and then smiled at me. "Let's wait for a bit on that and get this second Fast ForWord program under way."

I agreed and felt there was a plan. She'd given us a map, a navigator's tool, instead of our boat drifting aimlessly in a vast lavender ocean. A few minutes later, we left Gloria's office, having signed Ben up for Step 4word. Our insurance had denied the first program, and although Gloria's staff would bill our carrier, we weren't too optimistic about payment for the second program. We had to wait a few weeks for Gloria's office to get the CDs from Scientific Learning, and it was just as well, given Ben's school schedule.

I received Gloria's official report a few days later. Another envelope I didn't want to open. It reflected what Gloria had summarized: big gains made in the receptive scores, which were now "low–average," and lesser gains made in expression, which were still in the "extremely low range." Ben showed the most improvement in the Auditory Figure Ground (where background noise was present) subtest of the SCAN.

I laid the stapled packet down. The kids were at school, and the house seemed vacant, empty. Somehow I had thought we'd be further along, that the real world effects we'd witnessed with Fast ForWord would carry over a bit more into the test scores. But that wasn't what was bothering me. I knew the program had dramatically helped my son, and he was now able to perceive sounds in a new way. I just thought, hoped, yearned for someone to say, "You're done. He's okay now. You can all go on with your lives. It was enough."

* * *

FIRST GRADE. NOT REALLY THAT BIG A DEAL, I ASSURED MY-self. I'd arranged for Ben's teacher, Miss Rice, to meet with him a few times before school started so that she could get to know him, and he could get used to his new room. The sessions went well from what I could tell. His teacher had long straight hair. I could imagine first-grade girls pining after the long locks and little boys staring for different reasons. Miss Rice was young— in her twenties—not married, no children. Yet she carried authority in her bearing, and her lanky height added to the feeling that this was her room and when those kids were there, they belonged to her.

After first grade had been in session for a couple of weeks, I stopped by the school to do some parent volunteer work. The teachers left baskets of various tasks to be done, and I'd just picked up a folder of papers that needed to be copied. The copy machine just happened to be outside Ben's classroom. Suddenly, Miss Rice appeared next to me. She stopped hesitatingly, and I took the opportunity to describe Fast ForWord to her, but found it hard to explain the program.

"It's more than computer games. The program is based on auditory skills as well as language and processing language."

She raised an eyebrow in partial understanding.

"You download the data after each day, and the games adapt to the child's performance."

Another nod and both eyebrows rose.

"We're going to do the follow-up program." I hesitated. "How's Ben doing?"

"Okay, I think. I've just now got to the point that I can understand him for the most part. We'll see. First grade is pretty intensive." She flipped her hair back. "We're still trying to figure out how to best meet his needs." There was another first-grade teacher who split up the curriculum with Miss Rice. Miss Rice was in charge of language arts, while the other instructor was responsible for math.

I shifted my weight as I glanced inside the room, trying to see Ben. "Let me know if there's any way I can support him at home. I'm happy to reinforce anything that seems difficult for him."

"Thanks. I'll let you know. I've found that writing notes in his planner is a good way to communicate with parents. Just write a note if you have questions or anything." A flash of straight white teeth.

"Okay. I'll be sure to check it."

After a bit more chat, I said good-bye to Miss Rice, and put another paper inside the copy machine. My memory of Ben's meltdown in front of her last February was still vivid. I kept thinking there was a clock ticking in a countdown to Ben's time at the school, and Miss Rice would announce one day that the alarm had gone off, and we were out.

BEN HAD DAILY HOMEWORK THAT TOOK US ANYWHERE FROM a half hour to two hours a night. The student planner that Miss Rice had mentioned also helped him to keep track of his assignments. He had a "book in a bag" due weekly, which included short books to read with activity cards and written assignments. The exercises on the cards ranged from alphabetizing words to grouping words by sounds. There were also weekly spelling words to memorize and math booklets. Addition and subtraction were two of Ben's strong skills. Finally, the children were expected to learn and practice cursive writing. I thanked God for every minute Elizabeth had spent with him working on his fine motor strength and control.

I was still in regular contact with Gloria, who had just received the second Fast ForWord program, Step 4word. The cost was about the same as the first program. But as one of the first families to use the program, we received a small discount of about a hundred and fifty dollars. I wrote Gloria one night in mid-October:

Ben got 100% on his math test and cut his time (they time the kids) by half! Can you believe it? He is also making the adjustment to first

grade in that he is able to tell me his feelings that are changing from sad-
ness to irritation to sometimes justified anger. He is also—and this is a
biggie—able to verbally tell me what happened at school that day. For
example, a boy took candy from one of the girls; the teachers had difficulty
keeping the kids quiet, etc. And he is making new friends, mostly with
girls. Spelling and phonics are still lagging, but that's why we're doing
the next program. Karen.

Lagging was probably too mild a word to use. Ben received a
zero on his first spelling tests. He wasn't able to write even a
guess at the letters. I studied one of his sheets and saw a pathetic
scrawl as he attempted to write the first word. Then no more
tries. A blank sheet of paper. Simple words such as "bat," "tab,"
"see," "bus," "sit," and "us" were still impossible for him. I was
more than ready to begin Step4word on October 21.

Unlike during the summer when I didn't have to drive anywhere, be anyplace at a certain time, or adhere to any schedule,
Step 4word was going to have to be fit in after a full day of school
at least three days a week. Not easy, particularly when homework
would also need to be done.

Gloria e-mailed me the access numbers for us to begin play.
Ben sat down willingly, and I let Peter play with some toys in the
basement so that he could be nearby—as long as he promised to
be quiet.

The graphics were much improved over the first program.
There were five games now, instead of seven: Start-Up Stories
(SS), Treasure in the Tomb (TT), Trog Walkers (TW), Polar Cop
(PC), and Bug Out! (BO). This program allowed Ben to choose
the order of the games, which were played for eighteen minutes
instead of twenty as in the first program. That equaled ten minutes less playtime per night—a big deal when the child sitting
next to you is exhausted.

Start-Up Stories (SS) combined the language exercises, spatial
placement, and following oral directions. Two to four pictures appeared on the screen with one correct description and three dis-
tracters: Ben heard the voice say, "The duck that is chasing the

hen that is small, is big." One duck would be big, one small; one hen would be big, one small. In order for his answer to be counted correctly, Ben was expected to understand that the hen was small and the duck was big by choosing the correct picture.

Second, there were grids of sixteen objects with various tasks to complete. Ben was asked to place objects: "Put the small red crayon between the yellow sheep and the blue plane"; and follow directions: "Touch the small yellow gloves and the large red feather." Being adept at working, dragging, and clicking the mouse was crucial in this part of the game. I could see immediately that Ben had improved in his ability to follow oral directions.

A new, third component to SS was an exercise where the computer voice read short stories to the child, who was then asked to answer content/comprehension questions. Ben had difficulty with these questions, particularly when a lot of different characters' names were in the story.

The second game, Treasure in the Tomb (TT) was one of my favorites, perhaps because of my fascination with ancient Egyptian culture. Through completion of the exercises, a cat named Nephertari dug deeper and deeper into Pharaoh Phoneme's tomb. Ben was given a target word such as "bid." He saw the letters as well as heard them while two ancient Egyptian characters faced each other, one saying the target word, and the other a similar word that varied in the beginning or ending sound, such as "lid."

The third game, Polar Cop (PC), was particularly childlike and filled with humor. A polar bear, dressed as a policeman, was trying to find the words stolen by the penguins. Again, Ben was given a target word such as "gash," and similar words flashed on the screen while being spoken, such as "dash" and "cash." Sometimes he'd get impatient and click too soon or get confused with words that began with "b" and "d."

The fourth game was called Bug Out! and included fun characters as well. Dr. Insectus was trying to capture words. However, in Bug Out! entire words were uncovered by clicking on scarabs—like the tiles in Phonic Match in the first program. Ben was started with four scarabs, with two matching sets of words, and advanced to eight, then sixteen. The fewer clicks he used to match, the more points he could earn.

The last game, Trog Walkers (TW), was excruciating for Ben. Similar to Circus Sequence in the use of high/low sweeping tones, this game advanced from two to five consecutive tones, depending on the child's performance. Grandpa Lugnut explained that he had a time machine and would transport the player back to the "time of dinosaurs and cavemen and Trog Walkers." The better Ben played, the faster his caveman walked as measured by a speedometer on the screen.

We experienced a couple of days of technical problems—Polar Cop froze up and the sound disappeared on Trog Walkers. But the technical support at Scientific Learning helped John troubleshoot the difficulty. Still, it was unnerving to have the games suddenly stop. The downside to technology.

BEN'S WORKDAY DIDN'T END WHEN SCHOOL WAS OVER. IN fact, his second shift began with homework and Step 4word. Again, Ben worked very hard. Week Two's data were strong, with his scores averaging 20% across the games. By Week Four, the game scores started to spread out, indicating which ones were more challenging for him. Polar Cop (44%) and Trog Walkers (46%) lagged behind the other three. He'd jumped in Treasure in the Tomb (76%) and Bug Out! (75%). Start-Up Stories stood at a respectable 60% completion score.

One Thursday in late November, I arrived home at 3:45 P.M. with a tired Ben and Pete. They crashed through the door, dumped backpacks, shoes, and coats in the vicinity of where the items were supposed to go, and headed for the TV. I looked at the uncooked spaghetti I'd planned for dinner, wishing McDonald's delivered, and flipped through the pages of Ben's student planner. I discovered he had three pages of math and four pages of printing work to do that night. What might take another child a half hour to do, would take Ben at least two. To make matters worse, we were on Day Two of the Step 4word exercises.

I walked over to Ben and tried to get his attention away from "The Real Adventures of Johnny Quest." "Honey, we have a lot of homework tonight and Step 4word to do."

Ben's eyelids flickered, indicating he'd heard me.

A few minutes later, I'd managed to feed him and Peter a snack and coax Ben into the basement and sit him in front of the monitor. Gloria thought trying Trog Walkers first might help. It was his most challenging game. Ben stiffened as Grandpa Lugnut began his recitations at the start of the race.

"Come on, Ben." I glanced to where Peter was playing. "You can do it. Let's sit up and lean forward. Try to repeat the tones as you hear them."

He tried. Bless his heart, he tried so hard. Two were easy. Three tones made him think. On a good day, four were doable. Five were impossible.

I leaned forward and listened. "High/low/low/low/high."

Ben clicked the wrong sequence and the sound of failure—a dull metal thud—rang out. He angrily shoved the mouse away. "I hate this shitty Trog Walker game."

I sat there, not moving. I knew where he'd heard the word, and it wasn't John or school. After the initial shock began to wear off, I suppressed a giggle. I was an awful mother to laugh about this. But the sentence was grammatically correct, an adjective modifying a noun. All the components were there, and he'd expressed how he felt.

Suddenly, I realized he was staring at me, ready to cry. "Ben, you shouldn't use that word," I said lamely. "I know it's hard. Let's try to finish the games, okay?" I squeezed his hand.

"I know." He wiped his face and round brown eyes. "I sorry."

A few minutes later, after the other games were finished, I downloaded the data and called him over to me. "You know, you're my hero, Ben. Do you know what that means?"

He shook his head.

"It means you've worked really hard and that you're brave. You've done so much, Ben. You can listen so much better now. You're my hero because you try so very much." I held him in my arms.

He pulled away from my squeeze and seemed calmer.

I kissed him about ten times on his cheeks, and let Ben and Peter pick a small toy from the box. I waited for confirmation that his data had been received and stared into the computer screen, hearing the kids thump loudly into the kitchen upstairs.

It seemed like two lifetimes ago when I woke up in my bed alone before John was in my life, before the kids. I'd take an hour to curl my hair, sip my tea, and apply my makeup. I even ironed my clothes back then. Yet, when I stared into the mirror, I liked what was inside me now more than during my single days. I'd grown more tolerant of others, less judgmental, more apt to listen to others' feelings. Less self-involved.

And I loved, but also liked, my children. I admired Ben and liked being with him. His personality spoke of characteristics born out of struggles: He had great empathy toward other children. Miss Mary would stop me to tell me how kind Ben had been to a classmate who had been stung by a bee. He'd get upset if Peter cried. He'd never been unkind toward his brother—not in any aggressive or mean-spirited way. In fact, because there were no neighborhood kids to play with, the brothers played for hours together.

Peter pushed me some days with his endless nags. But if I looked a little deeper, I knew him to be a kind and sincere boy. He made me laugh. They were so different in temperament. Ben was laid-back and easygoing. Quiet and reserved. A person who could stay at home his whole life and be content. Peter was verbally skilled and inquisitive.

When I'd buy each of the boys a toy during a Wal-Mart run, I'd usually let them hold them in the car. Within seconds, Peter would rip the package apart, lose five of the smallest pieces, and unbuckle himself to look for them. Ben would sit silently, examining the toy through the clear plastic and deciding he would wait to open it when he got home for fear of losing any of the parts.

I heard the boys getting into the chips and knew I'd better get upstairs. The computer message told me that data had been successfully downloaded. I switched it off and vowed to swear less frequently.

SOMETHING WAS HAPPENING AS STEP 4WORD CONTINUED. Ben's spelling tests at school showed marked improvement. By December, he was able to get 100% on 18-word spelling tests. His performance wasn't consistent, but he was able to write the words as they were spoken. His parent/teacher conference reflected more gains, which I shared with Gloria:

We had Ben's conference yesterday, and it went pretty well. What I heard the teachers wanting to know was if they were approaching Ben's learning needs in the most efficient ways possible. They seemed to be relieved when we expanded on John's history of learning differences. Ben's ability to spell and his reading skills are quickly expanding. He's actually excited to participate in the spelling group. His math skills are good. Socially he fits in well. They did say he "often responds inappropriately—out of context—to questions." I think that they mean he's on another topic or doesn't directly answer their questions. Honestly, John and I don't pick up on this at home, but maybe we know him so well, we know what he's referring to. They admitted he was often excited when he did this or in a group setting where there is pressure on him to perform. They did say his expressive gains had been significant this year. They mentioned more speech and hearing testing, but I deferred to you and was wondering if you could either talk to Ben's teachers or outline a simple list of suggestions for communicating with him (classroom interventions). Thanks, Karen.

Gloria was able to contact Miss Rice and his other teacher. Both teachers reported this was helpful in understanding Ben's needs. They also reported Ben had difficulty recognizing the letters b, d, p, and q—a skill worked on in Polar Cop, one of Ben's harder games. I continued to get the feeling that, despite how much I liked the school and appreciated the teachers' efforts to help Ben, the resources he needed weren't there.

We'd stopped having the private speech therapist come to the house last spring before the first Fast ForWord program. (Both programs had now been denied by our insurance company.) Because speech therapy wasn't available at the Montessori school and because the Fast ForWord programs were so intense, Ben wasn't receiving any direct work on his expression. I began to look seriously at the fit between the school and my son. That tick-tock was growing louder. And so on a gloomy late November day, I decided to visit the local school that was just a six-minute drive from our house.

The school reminded me of a typical small town school. It wasn't too big, with an enrollment of about 300 kids, but it was large enough to give kids a choice of friends. It was a flat, light-red brick building with long parking spaces out front for the buses to load the kids at the end of the day. A flagpole just outside the front entrance boasted the American and Indiana State flags. These symbols perhaps spoke the most strongly to me. It was a public school. Inclusive. Funded by citizens through taxation. And with bureaucratic federal and state educational laws to uphold.

I parked the car, and tried to breathe more evenly. Inside the front glass doors, the cream-colored cement brick walls were lined with student artwork. A small suite of administrative offices held a sign marked, "All Visitors Must Check in at the Front Office." A middle-aged woman with dark short hair twirled in her chair as she went from answering the phone, sending brief messages over the intercom, and handing notes to people passing by. This was a pro, and I figured she'd been at this job for years.

"Yes?" Her eyes peered at me from above her glasses.

"I'm the mother of a first-grade little boy—he doesn't go here. But we live here in town. He goes to the Montessori school down the road. And, well, I was wondering if I might," I stuttered, "look, look around."

A quick once-over. "I'll see if our principal, Mr. Franklin, can chat with you for a few minutes."

I waited for a short time and was greeted by a white-haired elderly gentleman who impressed me as a person waiting eagerly for retirement—which the local paper said was imminent. He was cordial and told me that they had all of the services, like speech, that Ben might need. His relaxed demeanor was emphasized by his slouch in the chair. After a brief conversation, he stood up, escorted me back to the secretary's desk, and invited me to, "Have a look around. The second-grade teacher rooms are just down the hall, to your right."

I looked back just in time to see him disappear into his office.

After pinning my visitor badge on, I crept down the corridor. It seemed so much bigger than the Montessori school. Would Ben get lost? I turned and started to look for the signs outside the doors that marked the teacher and grade. I peeked inside a room and a blond-haired woman in her mid-fifties smiled at me. "Can I help you?"

Her voice was like oral Calgon, almost lyrical, but with an underlying firmness to it. "Boys and girls, get your pictures out, your glue and scissors." She turned back to the room for an instant to make sure the kids complied. I know I would have if I'd been at a desk.

After noting that this was Mrs. Perkins's second-grade class, I stepped into the room. "I'm just here to look around. I have a little boy in first grade, and I wanted to visit the school. I'm thinking of bringing him here next year." My fingers absently went to the visitor badge on my chest. "I don't want to disturb your class."

"No. Come on in." She waved me inside, and the twenty-some boys and girls turned from their desks, which were in five straight lines, to examine the stranger entering their turf. Mrs. Perkins, with one arm around my shoulders and her face toward the class, said, "Boys and girls, I want you to finish your projects quietly while I speak with our guest."

Mrs. Perkins's hair reached her shoulders, and she wore a denim jumper complete with red apple patch on each pocket. It reminded me of what a teacher was supposed to wear. She was im-maculately groomed and met me with clear eyes. This was a teacher kids remembered for years.

She showed me a seat beside her desk, but I remained stand-ing, sure I would only be there for a few more minutes. "Now, how can I help you?"

"My name is Mrs. Thompson and my little boy is at the Montessori school, but I was wondering if perhaps he shouldn't come here next year. He's got some speech problems and needs help with hearing things sometimes. He's not what you'd call a strong reader."

She pulled the chair a bit closer to me. This time I sat down. She told me she was finishing her third decade of teaching. That speech therapy was available. The average class size was around twenty-five. I asked if it was a safe school, and she replied that it was. Taunting, name-calling, and physical aggressiveness weren't tolerated. It wasn't unusual for children to come to second grade not being able to read. She could tell me stories about kids who caught up just fine. Now, mind you, she had to work a little harder with them, but that was all right.

Suddenly, for no reason, I felt like crying. She was so kind and helpful. Could I finally allow the system to help me? No more tick-tock. No more asking what to do next for him. Someone to help make it enough.

She must have seen me struggling, because she stood up to show me around the room, explaining the work the children were doing, how the class was organized. I left a half hour later, torn and relieved. Little did I know that this woman would play an important role in Ben's future.

OFFICIALLY, BEN COMPLETED THE EIGHT-WEEK PROGRAM OF Step 4word on December 11. His scores reflected the hours and hours of hard work: Treasure in the Tomb, Start-Up Stories, Polar

Cop, and Bug Out! were all over 90% completed. However, it was clear he'd not mastered Trog Walkers (70%). Gloria offered us the option of continuing to play *only* Trog Walkers. She instructed us to take a week off and then have him play over the Christmas break. John and I were in total agreement and were happy with the flexibility Gloria was showing us.

Ben played Trog Walkers for an additional three weeks. Although he'd shown steady progress throughout the program, his scores leveled off between 68% and 72%. While disappointed that he wasn't able to process the tones efficiently, I couldn't help but think that this little boy was getting tired, very tired.

On a cold day in mid-January, we drove north to Gloria's office for Ben's post-Step 4word testing. This time, it didn't seem quite so stressful, although I hated these testing sessions. It wasn't so much that I disagreed with what was concluded—although I did disagree with some of the statements on nearly every test report I'd ever read. It was that it carried so much power, to use words with such authority, and create a picture of a little boy that didn't reflect the Ben I knew.

The same tests were performed as after the first Fast ForWord program. As scored by the Test of Auditory Perceptual Skills (TAPS-R), Ben showed a significant gain from prior to *both* programs, but the test results still showed Ben in the "moderately low range." The Clinical Evaluation of Language Fundamentals (CELF-3) showed more dramatic improvements as Ben now scored in the average range. Ben's APD was so severe before starting the exercises; he was unable to do the Lindamood Auditory Conceptualization or LAC test. Now, he scored in the tenth percentile for children entering first grade. Overall, Ben gained twenty months in his language skills, although his expressive skills were still severely delayed.

The SCAN tests showed dramatic improvement in two of its three subtests. Filtered Words and Auditory Figure Ground subtests were now in the high average range. His Competing Words subtest remained in the low average range, although the SCAN composite score placed him in the high average range. Gloria concluded that his reading skills, while progressing, were still below those of his peers.

"I think you should do two things," Gloria said to John and me as we sat in her office, now a familiar place. "First, the *Fokes Sentence Builder* program would be helpful in building Ben's grammar and sentence formulation and second, the Lindamood-Bell LiPS program."

I looked at her, eager to learn, anxious to understand what she was referring to. "The Fokes program—that's what we talked about this fall, right?"

"Yes. It'd be perfect for Ben. It's very structured where you literally build the sentences with the child. You lay out cards labeled 'who,' 'is doing,' 'what,' and so on. With these cards, you make sentences. Like 'the teacher is writing on the blackboard.' Then, the child can read them to you. You build on the sentences, and the child learns to manipulate the different parts. But we'll start with the basics."

I nodded. "And you can order it for me?"

"Yes. I'll have them ship it directly to you. I'll have my staff member let you know how much it is, and you can pay my office."

"Thanks. I've heard of Lindamood-Bell. The lady, the mom, who told me about Fast ForWord also mentioned she did the program for her daughter."

Gloria's eyes opened wider, and I could almost see them sparkle. "It's great stuff. I can bring you up here for training, if you'd like. Since you're so far away, that might be the best."

"How long does it take to learn the program?"

"About two weeks. Not that long." She stood up and turned toward Ben, who kept saying, "Go home now?"

"Yes, Ben. We're all done. Can I get a hug?"

Ben awkwardly put his arms around her, and I noticed how he wasn't too much shorter than the petite woman. Gloria smiled, shook John's hand, then mine and bid us good-bye.

*   *   *

THE WRITTEN REPORT THAT FOLLOWED A FEW DAYS LATER was much as before. Aside from the summary of test findings, there were comments about Ben's eye contact or lack thereof, a recommendation for sensory integration therapy, and an intellectual assessment. I tossed it aside, tired of it all, knowing that it wasn't entirely accurate and worrying that deep down, my assessment of Ben might not be, either.

I clutched my children inside the boat, and looked over the side to see that the lavender water was a bit lighter than before. The shoreline was now more visible, a clear outline in the distance. But the water had stilled, and in order to move forward at all, I had to row the boat. I rowed steadily, as if on autopilot, ignoring the cramps in my muscles and the exhaustion in my head and wondering if and when I could stop. When would it be enough?

CHAPTER TWELVE

Feeling Sound

GLORIA HAD MENTIONED BEN NEEDED MORE SENSORY INTE-
gration therapy. With this in mind, the four of us drove to Indianapolis on New Year's Eve to purchase a scratched and dented
aboveground pool for the summer. Ben was a natural swimmer.
Never having taken lessons, he had taught himself how to navigate
the water. And Peter was old enough now to enjoy a larger pool.

I hoped that I'd feel a renewed energy when both of the Fast
ForWord programs were finished. That Ben, now almost seven
years old, would dive into school with renewed vigor. But it
didn't happen. Instead, it was more of a chore getting him to concentrate. While his home-based tutor, Jamie, reported great
progress overall, his performance was inconsistent. I couldn't remember him laughing anymore—not the whole body, belly-
shaking laughs that I loved.

The kids at school, whose verbal skills far surpassed his, tended
to play games with him, not exactly taunting, but not exactly fair
either. Ben would report that one of his classmates would tell
him, "I'm your friend." Then the next minute, "No. I'm not your
friend." From "I'll play with you" to "No. I won't play with you."
Ben would get into the car at the end of the day, bewildered. I
could see defensiveness in his eyes. And by Friday afternoon,

some oppositional behaviors. He answered simple requests with "I don't want to." He showed regressive behaviors, crying easily when frustrated or angry. I also began to see the signs of depression in Ben. A malaise. A flatness inside him.

On a damp winter day around Valentine's Day, I looked out of the bedroom window to see Ben lying on the cold asphalt of our drive with his arm around Sheldon, our Shetland sheepdog. Ben stared at the clouds, not moving, and as I inched closer to the window, I thought I saw him wipe his cheek.

I spoke to John about it, and he'd noticed the change in Ben, too. We agreed to lighten up on any pressure academically. What he could do, he could do.

My guilt toward Peter waxed and waned. I felt good about how he thrived at the Montessori school and drove to the school early one morning to help him celebrate his half-birthday. Mrs. Minett, his teacher now for two years, measured the paper crown carefully, stapled it in place, and coronated Peter "King for the Day." Peter adored Mrs. Minett and the attention. Today he was at the height of his glory.

A tiny girl with almost white hair plunked down on my lap. Her blue eyes looked at mine and then she lay back, curling into my well-padded lap. I tingled and ached. Another child. A girl, this time. What I wouldn't give to have it all back. The baby years. I watched my little boy, now four and a half, and grieved for all his lost baby years, when I was so immersed in Ben. I thought of Halley, the psychic, and her prediction of another child. But no, it wasn't possible for John and me. We had too much going on.

Mrs. Minett presented Peter to the class, and just before I snapped his picture, I gently took the little girl off my lap and clapped loudly for Peter.

A FEW DAYS AFTER HIS HALF-BIRTHDAY PARTY, I DECIDED TO take Peter on a special outing. "Peter, we're just going to look today, all right?" I tried to catch his eye as I drove down the highway a short distance from our home.

He squirmed in his seat, nodded, and laughed without cause. "We're just going to pet them. *No dog* today." He giggled again, and I knew he didn't believe a word he and I were saying.

"Just pet." He waited a bit. "What are we going to call the puppy?"

"Pete! We're just going to see if we can volunteer to pet the doggies once in a while."

We arrived at the Humane Society building, a run-down house that somebody had probably donated long ago. A couple of cars were parked in the gravel lot as I pulled up. What the hell was I doing? Another thing to take care of? Our dog population had increased to four—almost pack size—due to a stray that'd been dumped the previous spring. Bud, as we called him, was one smart dog, having survived months on his own. Someone had taken the time to toilet-train him and teach him to shake paws. The vet had treated his intestinal worms, vaccinated him, and neutered him. We'd tried to take him to the shelter, but at the time, they didn't have any space. Now a plump black and white Spaniel mix, he knew where home was.

So here I was today, looking for what? What was it inside me that couldn't just leave it alone? Why did I feel like everything around me was dormant or dead? Just because a little girl sat on my lap, did that mean a puppy would fix that longing? Or make Ben laugh again? This is what I got for reading the local paper and seeing all the new abandoned puppies.

I went around the other side of the van to help Peter down. "Just look and pet," I repeated.

Peter shot his hand out and very adult-like flattened it in the air. "Just look."

The odor of penned-up animals hit us immediately as we opened the door, a mixture of animal waste and chlorine bleach. From behind a closed door, barks and loud meows, and growls intermingled into a frenzy. A tired-looking woman with limp shoulder-length hair greeted us with as much of a smile as I guessed she was capable of. "Can I help you?"

"I saw the ad where you had some Golden Retriever puppies that were dumped."

"Yes. We have quite a few at the moment. There's about two or three from each of the litters we got, I'd guess." She nodded to a teenage girl who appeared in the doorway. "Go get the Retriever pups."

"The Labs?"

"No. The Goldens." She disappeared through a door that when opened let out a cacophony of canine howls.

I looked at Peter. His face was pale and his mouth was no longer smiling. His eyes darted around, trying to peer down the hallway where the girl had gone. "It's okay. Do you want to leave?" I whispered.

"No. It stinks in here."

I nodded just before the girl reappeared with about five small dogs on leashes. There, right at the end, was a little female puppy, with a face that put any stuffed animal imitation to shame. Her coat was a fuzzy yellow; her short ears flopped as she strained at the leash. She looked at me, and the naked fear in her eyes pulled at me.

"Pete. Look at that one." I pointed. "At the end."

Peter walked over, knowing no trepidation from animals. He bent down to pet her.

"Is she a Golden?" I asked the lady.

"Who knows?" She puffed at her cigarette and came from around her gray metal desk to look at the pup. With one hand, the lady scooped up the little dog's face. "She looks it."

Peter turned his head up from the puppy. "Can we have her, Mom?"

"Is she due to, you know, to be—"

"She's past her time. She's been here over two weeks. We usually have the doctor put them down sooner than that."

I took a breath and thought what a deep-down mess of contradictions I was, but I didn't have time to sort through them all at that moment. "Okay. Is there paperwork?"

"Just a form or two." She shrugged. "You can take her today. We're so full, it'd help us out."

I swallowed. "Sure." And watched Peter give me a smile as he gently petted the frightened puppy.

After filling out some biographical information and writing a check, and receiving a card for free spaying at the local veterinarian's office, I loaded Peter and now a puppy into the van. My boy's face was in a radiant smile, and he couldn't take his eyes off the little fur ball in his possession. It struck me how loving his little hands were, how soft his voice was, trying to reassure this abandoned life that he would make sure she was okay. What a treasure this little boy of mine was.

A few hours later, John and Ben came home to a new puppy, which had christened our carpet with Number One and Number Two. John, who loved animals and kids, was delighted with our addition. I watched closely after Ben walked into the living room and saw the puppy for the first time.

Ben's hand reached out and stroked the fur. He kept stroking and stroking, as if he couldn't get enough. The puppy danced around, pulling at her chew toy, falling sideways, and then I heard a long ago laugh reappear. His giggle turned into a full tummy rumble. Words were interspersed with his giggles, "No. Oh, no. Look, Peeda."

John crossed his arms, smirking at me, knowing me so well and yet never interfering with who I needed to be. "What's her name?"

I turned to stir the chili soup. "How about Kanga? She's the only female character in the Pooh series, with the exception of Christopher Robin's mother, whose face we've never seen."

John had added an outright twinkle in his eye to his smirk. "Okay."

"And I thought we needed some more female energy in this house, you know?"

John stopped after setting the water glasses on the table.

I put the lid back on the saucepan. "Remember about a week ago, I told you about the little girl who sat on my lap?

Well, I can't quit thinking about it. What would you think about adopting a little girl? I know we've both thought about adoption before we met. It's not something entirely new to either of us." My words ran into each other. Scared to come out of me.

"That'd be okay. I'd like a little girl."

He'd said it so evenly. Like I'd just finished a weather report. "I'm serious, John."

"Me, too."

It was then I noticed that he was very serious.

I took a breath, wiped the stovetop with a damp rag, and blurted, "Have you ever thought that maybe—maybe—you do have some auditory problems? Maybe Ben did get them from you. I don't know." I checked John's expression. He seemed to be okay with what I was suggesting. "Think about it. How many times have you misunderstood what I've said to you? How many times have you come home from a meeting and told me, 'I need time to process what went on'?"

John looked directly at me. "I know. I've thought about it as well. I guess I might have it. Maybe that's why I understand Ben so well. But some of it doesn't make sense. I like having things read to me more than reading it, especially when I'm tired."

I checked the cornbread baking in the oven. We'd had Gloria's staff check John's hearing at Ben's last visit. His hearing acuity was normal.

I continued, "I agree. Some of it's like Ben and some of it's totally different. How do you feel about it?"

He sat down at the table and met my eyes from across the kitchen island. "I'm not sure. I knew in med school that fast-paced, noisy places weren't for me. That's why I knew I didn't want to work in intensive care or the emergency room where information has to be processed so quickly. I knew I needed a slower pace."

"Like psychiatry," I said.

"Yeah. Come to think of it, I've always used the patient's non-verbal stuff when I do therapy. I get a lot of information that way."

I leaned forward. "Noisy restaurants are really hard places for you. When we're in a place with a lot of background noise, you just can't seem to hear me. And maybe it's somehow linked to your bumpy rides with the past jobs . . ."

"Maybe so." He'd grown quiet and stared at the table.

I went over and rubbed his back. I wanted to let him know it was all right. I struggled to keep my voice even, to get this out once and for all. "And you know, I guess if we did adopt, it would help me get over this sense of loss and blame. It has no rational basis. It's selfish, but I feel it sometimes. I mean, you've learned how to cope. You're so good at what you do and all." My voice cracked. "And I want another baby. I can't explain it."

John stood up and held me. "I think we should adopt. It's okay." And he continued to hold me while I started to weep and tell him I was sorry.

The boys and puppy came running into the room, so I wiped my face hurriedly. Satisfied the food was cooked, I started to take the cornbread out of the oven and glanced at the boys playing with the puppy. "Come on, boys, let's eat." I turned to John, whose look of concern made me understand why I loved him so much. "We can talk about it later. I wouldn't want to do anything that would hurt the boys."

"Nah. They're fine."

"And I'm pushing forty."

"You look great."

That was my John.

A FEW WEEKS LATER, I SCHEDULED BEN'S LAST PARENT-teacher conference. Miss Rice and her colleague had really gone the extra mile with Ben. But aside from his fatigue after the Fast ForWord programs, Ben had hit a plateau in his reading, spelling, and writing. He wrote his name, "Ben Thomen." His phonetic abilities, after two years of phonics work, seemed impaired and imprecise. His ability to write words was also clearly scrambled: "redeng" was "reading." At the end of the term, he was asked to answer, "What my portfolio shows about my writing." He answered, "alrallanraneg." I truly couldn't guess at what he was trying to say.

Ben didn't seem able to put vowels into words or divide words. By the end of first grade, his spelling tests had begun to include more difficult words. His ability to discriminate between sounds, particularly vowel sounds, made for many spelling errors: hav/have; hem/him; met/mitt; fet/fit; wel/will; sken/skin; tek/tack; pad/band.

A few days prior to the conference, Miss Rice had arranged for the first-graders to meet with their second-grade teachers. Unlike the traumatic episode of last year, Ben handled the visit well. They quoted him in the class newsletter: "I think second grade will be fun. I will have a nice day. Second grade is easy. I will have a nice day with my new teacher."

A milestone had passed for me. I told John I could solo this conference. He had a particularly busy day of patients, and I felt I could handle it on my own. Still, my hands told me how nervous I was, and as I sat down facing Miss Rice, I wasn't sure the tick-tock had stopped completely.

Miss Rice started with compliments about Ben. "Ben stays on task and treats others with respect. He also follows class rules."

The other teacher added, "I think one of Ben's strengths is math computation. This might be an area where he could really excel."

Back to Miss Rice. "I think, while Ben has some issues he needs to continue to work on, he's okay to move on to second grade. We can understand him so much more. He has a great sense of humor and is able to have friends and play on the playground."

We finished the conference, and I thanked them both profusely. As I walked to the car, I tried hard to understand exactly where Ben fell. He'd passed first grade without being able to write clear sentences or read at his age level. But I didn't want him held back and didn't think that he should be. The school

didn't give grades, just detailed feedback on the child's performance, and I knew the boy who had arrived at their classroom
last fall was far different than Ben today. But I couldn't help but
compare him to the children in his class who could write poems,
do simple multiplication, and whose verbal skills far surpassed
Ben's. He wasn't getting speech therapy and Gloria said he'd need
that.

I turned the key to start the car and pulled out of the parking
lot. My foot pushed on the gas pedal. Just as the fuel enabled the
car to accelerate, a surge of pride energized me. Ben had defused
the bomb. No more ticking sounds.

Yes, Ben was safe at this school. Peter was thriving under Mrs.
Minett's care. I hated to split the boys up. I had to consider Peter
now as well. The student–teacher ratio was much lower than that
quoted to me by Mrs. Perkins, the public school teacher I'd spoken with in the fall. Ben needed as much one-on-one attention as
he could get. I shoved my feelings of hesitation and unease aside
and gave myself permission—for this moment at least—to replay
again and again the positive things that were said about my child
today.

After basking in Ben's victory conference, I decided that if I
was going to keep Ben at the Montessori school, I needed to do
more. I just didn't know what that was. My question of whether
or not what we'd done was enough was answered by yes and no.
He was functioning—barely—at grade level, but his expressive
skills, his language skills in reading and spelling, and his social
skills were still lacking. Feelings of inadequacy plagued me as I
tried to work with Ben on the *Fokes Sentence Builder* program.
Gloria had said to start with "who is doing what" type sentences.

"Come on, Ben." I laid the black plastic board on the table and
placed the piles of cards marked "who," "is doing," and "what"
above it.

He looked at me. "I hate this."

"I know. Let's just give it a try." I picked the card that said,
"The boy" from the "who" pile, the card that said, "is riding"

from the "is doing" pile, and the card that said "the bike" from the "what" pile. "Okay." I pointed to the sentence. "The boy is riding the bike." I exhaled, sensing major resistance.

Silence.

"You say it, Ben."

"The boy is riding the bikes." His head tilted back and forth in a singsong obnoxious way.

"The bike. Just one."

"The bike." His teeth were tightly closed as he spoke.

"You make up one now."

He picked up the cards and threw a few down, not really caring if they were in the right order. We plodded through a few more sentences. There was something else I was missing. And as my eyes examined his curly brown hair, his little glasses, his full lips, now in a pout, I vacillated between feeling joy at his progress this year and the gap between Ben and his peers in language. It wasn't enough.

IT WAS NEARLY APRIL, AND MY MIND KEPT THINKING ABOUT the mother whose kindness had opened the door to finding Gloria and the Fast ForWord programs. I decided not enough people said "thank you" these days and wanted to tell her how much she had helped me. I fished out my address book and looked up her name—I knew her only by her first name.

"Hello?" I recognized her voice, a slow, deliberate, intelligent voice, and reintroduced myself.

"I just wanted to say thank you for the information you shared with me last spring—I guess it's been about a year. We ended up doing both Fast ForWord programs, and they helped Ben, my son, a lot."

"You know this is so weird because I was just thinking about you, too. I tried to find your number, but I couldn't, so I'm glad you called. I just got a brochure from the lady who taught me Lindamood-Bell. She's going to have another one on the LiPS program. Would you like me to send you the information?"

"Oh, that'd be great." I sat down. It was more than I'd hoped for.

"Let me see. Yes, here's the flyer. The lady who's giving it is really good. You know, it's in a few weeks." A pause. "Maybe I'd better give you her number in case you want to call her directly."

My hands pushed the calendar and phone books aside roughly as I tried to feel for a pen. I found one and ripped a scrap piece of paper off the pad. "Okay."

She read me the information, including the price, which seemed more than reasonable, about the cost of half a dozen speech therapy sessions. She ended with, "The LiPS seminar is a week-long course."

"Is it hard?"

A pause. "Not really. There's also V/V—she's doing that one in July."

"What's that?"

"The LiPS is for phonemic awareness—breaking down the sounds into phonemes. V/V or Visualization/Verbalization is more for reading comprehension and speech issues."

I lifted the pen up. Ben needed all of it. "You said before that it really helped your daughter."

"Definitely. They're great programs, and Zina, the lady giving the seminars, is really good at explaining it."

I continued to thank her until I sounded like someone strumming the same guitar string over and over. The last thing I wanted to do was to annoy, but it seemed to me the words inadequately expressed how much she'd helped.

THE NEXT DAY, I CALLED ZINA AND LEFT A MESSAGE FOR HER to call me. I explained on her voice-mail who I was and what I wanted. She called me back later that night.

"Yes. Thanks for returning my call. I'm interested in signing up for the LiPS program. I talked to one of your former students, and she gave me this information."

"Okay. I have to ask before we go any further, do you have any issues yourself?" Her voice had a lilt to it, like one who sang in the theater.

' I shooed Peter out of the bedroom—he had radar for when I was on the phone. I started to say my issues included occasional overeating and craving a cigarette once in a while. Instead, I said, "I'm not sure what you mean."

"I guess I wasn't very clear." I sensed a smile over the phone. "I mean, do you have any difficulty with reading or writing? Was school difficult in these areas for you? Have you ever been diagnosed with a learning difference? Or dyslexia? Because if you have, this will be very, very difficult for you to learn."

"No. It's my husband's fault," I said quickly and irreverently. I sensed a danger of being somehow disqualified. "Not to be arrogant, but all those areas came naturally to me. That's not to say I didn't work hard."

"Okay. It's just that I had a couple of ladies once who didn't tell me they'd had difficulties, and it was a really hard seminar for everyone."

"What kind of students do you have?"

"We don't have many moms learning the program, although I have a few. Mostly teachers and my students who help me with my tutoring. But I have to be careful with parents and others who show interest in my classes. For their sakes. I don't want them to waste their money."

"Are there any Lindamood-Bell Learning Centers in the state of Indiana?" For a moment, I thought how nice it would be to have Ben go to someone already trained in the techniques.

"No. Not now. I think there are plans to open one in a year or so."

"So, I can register for the class, right?" I felt shaky and was ready to plead yet again for a chance to help my son.

"You should be okay."

"Do you still have openings?" I held my breath.

A millisecond pause. "Yes. I think so. I'll write your name

down and send you a flyer with a registration form in it. Send it back as soon as possible."

I exhaled. "I look forward to receiving it."

IN ORDER TO ATTEND THE LIPS SEMINAR, I HAD TO MAKE strategic plans to have somebody pick up Ben and Peter, bring them home, and watch them until either John or I got home. A lady who was expecting her first child in October and who had worked at the Montessori day-care helped me out. She exuded freedom of spirit and a general satisfaction with life. She was a vegetarian and was one of those people who really did glow with the new life inside her.

Satisfied the boys were in good hands, I set out on a humid April day at six A.M. The dogs, all five, slept on the grass, their stomachs full from breakfasts.

"Yeah. Go ahead, you guys. Take it easy," I said. Kanga opened one eye and walked over to me. She'd grown into a young dog with beautiful colorings and a gentle personality. I briefly petted her before stepping into the car. I cranked the stereo to one of my favorite rock stations in Indy, drifting back to when I was on my own and living in the city. After two and a half hours, I neared the private school where Zina worked in support services.

My mind was caught up with what would be presented that day. I assumed that the program I was about to learn must rely heavily on visual cues. I reasoned that because the learner had auditory difficulties, the program must help compensate by building on visual strengths. I couldn't have been more wrong.

Once inside the building, a typical elementary school, although much nicer and bigger than the Montessori school, I followed the signs to where the seminar would be held. I recognized Zina's voice around a corner and stepped inside a classroom with clusters of tables seating four.

There were about half a dozen people already present, a mix of college students and a middle-aged lady with dark short hair.

They briefly smiled toward me before their attention was drawn once again to the table displaying bagels, pastries, and fresh coffee. I stiffly walked over to grab a Styrofoam cup, hoping the coffee was strong, when I heard a woman address me.

"Are you Karen Foli?"

"Yes."

"I'm Zina Northland. I have your LiPS manual up front. They just came in, thank goodness." She carefully picked up a cream cheese pastry and bit into it. "God, this is good." Her skin was dark, and her shiny coal black hair hung to her shoulders. Perhaps an Asian or Hawaiian heritage gave her such unique and beautiful features. The bodice of her colorful dress accentuated her petite frame, and her mannerisms made me think of a graceful young girl, although her face gave her an age of someone in her late forties.

Zina had walked to her table and picked up a heavy manual. With her free hand, she laid it next to my purse. The title read: *The Lindamood Phoneme Sequencing Program for Reading, Spelling, and Speech: The LiPS Program.* It was a thick, 8 ½- by 11-inch manual that Zina had ordered for me at the time I registered.

"Thanks." I added cream and sugar to my coffee. "How many folks are you expecting?"

"I think about eight in total. A couple of people canceled at the last minute. But it'll be a good group." She smiled and walked to the marker board and started to write.

Another woman, about my age, walked into the room, and my gut told me she was another mom. Maybe it was the fat purses we carried or our eyes that darted around tentatively. Or our short hair, designed to wash, dry, and hope for the best. She was slim and wore glasses and seemed to have a hard time not moving.

"Hi," I said.

"Hi," she answered as she reached for a coffee cup. We struck up a conversation, and I found out she lived in a neighboring city that I drove through on my way up to Indy. Before Zina asked us to take our seats, we'd already arranged to car pool the rest of the week. Fran told me she was married, had two kids, one girl in high school and a boy in third grade, and had recently moved from Illinois. There was something about her that reminded me of me.

"Okay," Zina started. "We're here to learn the LiPS program this week, which is a part of the Lindamood-Bell Learning Processes." She looked the group over. "Let's get started."

I got my pen out and opened the folder, expecting to be lectured to, the information fed to my auditorily intact system. It was not to be.

Zina positioned four different colored one-inch blocks in a straight line. She balanced them on a book and walked to the first student in the group. "Each of these blocks represents a different sound. I'm going to give you an old word and a new word. I want you to tell me the change and which block changes. This is called tracking chains." The student looked at her, somewhat hopelessly. I said a quick prayer of thank-you that I wasn't first.

Zina's smooth voice began, "If this is 'bink,' show me 'dink.'"

The student, a young man, who I assumed was one of the students whom Zina trained to tutor children, looked owlishly at the blocks. There was blue to represent b, yellow to represent the i, red for n, and white for k. "'Bink' to 'dink.' The first sound changes." She handed him a purple block, and he removed the blue block and placed the new block in front.

I took a long sip from my coffee, burning my tongue. Cheater, I thought childishly. I'll bet he's had some previous training.

Zina moved on to the next person, another young person, a woman, who didn't impress me as being as quick as the previous student. "If this is 'dink,' then give me 'denk.' I should tell you guys that the color isn't important. But know that if there is the same sound, then use the same colored block. So if it was 'sos,' the s's would be the same color. Okay. Let me start over." She let a moment of auditory silence fill the air. "'Dink' to 'denk.'"

The woman hesitated. My mind was blank. I longed to write something. To see something.

In a shaky, thin voice, the woman said, "'Dink' to 'denk.' The second sound changes."

"Good," Zina said. "The 'smile' vowels changed. We call it a 'smile vowel' because our mouth makes a smile when we make the sound." Her hands went to the sides of her mouth as she made the short "e" sound and a smile.

Then she went around the room to each student: "denk" to "delk" to "selk" to "selm" to my turn.

"Okay. If this is 'selm,' show me 'selch.'"

I sighed a breath of relief. "'Selm' to 'selch.' Change the final sound."

"That's right." She seemed pleased.

After a few more phonemic changes after "selch," which I didn't pay any attention to given my state of relief, Zina turned to the board to explain the interaction between auditory, visual, and language systems in comprehension. She explained how much we would cover, and I scoffed at learning so much in one short week. How could I possibly remember it all? Again, I was wrong.

I LEARNED A NEW WAY OF LEARNING, OF REGROUPING THE alphabet into sensory ways of feeling and hearing, and finally linking to a visual symbol. The first consonant pair we learned was the "p/b" pair or Lip Poppers.

Zina put a picture of a mouth on the board. Two lips slightly open with a small cloud of air coming from the mouth, as if it had just made the popping sound "p" or "b." Zina said, "'p.'"

"'puu,'" some of us said.

"No. Not 'puu.' Like this—'p,'" she repeated. "No 'u' sound at the end."

I did it as she instructed.

"Now 'b,'" she said. "This time, hold your hand over your throat."

A room full of hands clutched their throats.

"Feel that vibration?"

My fingers tingled as my larynx resonated inside me. Wow. It'd never occurred to me that my body did this when sounds were produced.

Zina continued. More pictures of the mouth forming sounds— no symbols or letters yet—just comparing and contrasting sounds. She went through the alphabet in a combination that was totally new and wonderful. After the first day, she'd finished the consonant letters that were paired together—Tip Tappers were "t/d"; Tongue Scrapers were "k/g"; Tongue Coolers were "th/*th*"; and so on. There were eight groups like this and eight more that were grouped by similarities in how the sounds were produced ("l/r" were Lifters). The vowel sounds were arranged in a circle that corresponded to how the mouth looked when making the sound (smiling, open, round). Then the physical sensation was linked to the sound heard.

My mind felt energized, feeling that familiar expansion as real learning takes place. As I picked up my purse and manual and prepared to leave for the day, my only question was how Ben would absorb this new information.

I COULD SEE FRAN, THE OTHER MOM AT THE SEMINAR, FROM across the room. She stood with her arms folded and her mouth closed in a firm, fixed line. I felt the tension and conflict in the room, and slowly walked closer to where Fran and a few others stood.

Fran said to a young woman standing across from her, "You don't know for sure, though, do you? Can you tell me with certainty that there wouldn't be consequences for blowing the whistle on my son's school?" Her voice shook under the strain of self-control. It was Day Four of the seminar, and we'd ridden together since Tuesday. She'd confided in me that her experiences with the local schools had been difficult. Her son hadn't been diagnosed with any specific learning problem, but she saw clear indications of struggle. Further, his performance and language test scores reflected a discrepancy, but one that the school refused to recognize.

She was speaking to Meg, who had short, blond hair and who wore loose jeans and torn shirts, but drove a nice car. Meg was a graduate student who was focusing on learning disabilities and had worked extensively with one little boy and his family.

Meg's voice was sure and confident. "I know that if you call the state department of education they have to take your complaint."

"And what about the repercussions? What about the possible backlash against my child?" Fran's nostrils flared. "I'm not willing to take that risk."

"What does the school say about your son?"

"They say he doesn't need any help. His grades are too good. But he tells me he forgets everything from one day to the next. Like somebody emptied his brain."

"You can get him help." Meg met Fran's eyes. The emotion in the room grew more intense. Zina had stepped out for a moment and a few others had left for lunch. It struck me how both women wanted the same thing, yet came from different perspectives. One, a mother, desperate to help her third-grade son, yet unwilling to draw political lines for fear of inciting the anger of the local school staff. She would rather pay for seminars like this one to try to help him at home. The other, a student, who was idealistic and zealous in her beliefs that the laws should be enforced to help all students, wanted to take on the system as an insider.

"They say the law ensures a 'free and appropriate' education. But I can tell you, Meg, it isn't that way." Fran went to grab her purse.

"You can call the state. It's the law."

Fran stood up tall, slung her purse over her shoulder, and crossed her arms. "Let me ask you this. If this was your child, and you'd already done everything you could to try to get him help, would you risk what you'd gained? Or would you come to seminars like this yourself to try to help him?"

Meg was silent. "I know it's hard. The system isn't perfect. There shouldn't be any repercussions to getting your child the help he needs."

Fran turned before she walked out the door. "But, believe me, I've seen these people in action, and it's a big risk."

I followed Fran out to her van and got into the passenger side.

Fran shook her head. "I shouldn't have said that. Meg's heart is in the right place. It's just different when it's your kid and you're the mom. There's no place else to send him. The school hates me. Thinks I'm an A Number-One Bitch." She sighed as she started the car. "Be glad you're not in the same county as I am."

I nodded silently as she kept on talking about her own purple water and how she'd been navigating it so far.

CHAPTER THIRTEEN

Down and Up

THE MONTH OF MAY MEANT THE END OF THE SCHOOL YEAR, and I was as ready to see it as Ben, now seven, was. We enrolled Ben for another year at the Montessori school, hoping the individual attention would continue to help his progress. Kanga had grown into a petite Golden Retriever, her fur the color of ripe apricots and as soft as down. We'd installed our aboveground pool, and as soon as it was warm enough, the boys jumped in.

The idea of another child wouldn't let go. I started to do research via the Internet and even called a few adoption agencies for their literature. But I'd been surprised and disappointed by people's reaction to our news of adopting. I'd heard a variety of responses:

"You've worked so hard with Ben. He still needs you. And Peter. It's not fair to them."

"You're no spring chicken, Karen. Babies are a lot of work."

"Why would you want to start over? Both boys will be in school full-time soon. Then you'll have all that time for yourself again."

John and I listened and despite being scared stiff, felt guided to adopt a baby. Obsessive Mom had taken over in many ways, and I didn't want her around any longer. For Ben's sake. For the family's sake. There was no question Ben was bright in his own way and could be very social. The Fast ForWord programs helped Ben to receptively understand what was said to him. It was now a question of how his reading and writing difficulties could be overcome, and Ben's expressive capabilities were still far below his peers. I continued to do research on auditory processing disorder and realized that it would never just go away. But armed with the knowledge from the LiPS seminar, I was eager to try the techniques with my oldest son.

I'd also ordered and received Earobics Step 2 and thought that given Ben's age, we could try that computer program along with the Lindamood-Bell. Jamie, Ben's tutor, was going to start coming again, about once a week. But I acknowledged that Ben needed some downtime, and Peter needed some time with me. Just to stay home. Just to be two little boys who knew nothing but the country life, collecting frogs, fishing, swimming, and relaxing.

Zina had shown us the materials we'd need to tutor others. Not much, really: small multicolored blocks; felt squares; a handheld mirror; small plastic letters; a pen and notebook; 3 $1/2$- by 5-inch index cards. I'd also copied the groups of letters and mouth pictures from the manual, which were supplied for that purpose. The pictures included the consonant pairs and vowel circle, and I covered them with a clear Con-Tact paper since I knew both Ben and I would be handling them frequently.

Lindamood-Bell was, at its very base, humanistic, one-on-one sensory stimulation. Just as Fast ForWord did something through a machine that no human could ever do, the LiPS program did something a machine could never do. The philosopher in me was fascinated with the contrast.

I decided to start LiPS with Ben after giving him the first two weeks of the summer off. I gathered up my supplies that fit into a standard-size plastic shoebox and called Ben upstairs. I decided to work at the desk I'd inherited from my great aunt Alda. She'd been an elementary-school teacher for decades before she retired.

It was a dark mahogany desk that brought back memories of her, a stoic woman who never married, who saw the Depression and the Wars, and lived a simple life by teaching children. I hoped good vibrations would come from the smooth surface as I began to arrange the first consonant picture.

Ben sat down, eyeing me. His stout solid legs stuck out awkwardly from the folding chair he was sitting on. The developmental height and weight charts couldn't plot his current husky build. His hair, now slightly highlighted due to the sun and pool, glimmered in the light. His round glasses accented his brown eyes. I gently pinched his chubby warm finger, something I did often.

"Ben, remember when Mommy went to school just before your school was out?"

He looked at me with a blank stare.

"Where I was a student for a week and sat at a desk?"

"Oh, yeah. Yeah."

"Well, I want to share with you what I learned. We're going to do a little of this every day, and then after we're done with the letters and sounds, we're going to read from a book."

He put his hands up to his eyes. "No. I don't want to read. It's hard."

"I think this will make it easier, Ben."

He moved his hands to look at me.

Without waiting for him to change his mind, I started. "Okay, I want you to make this sound for me, Ben: 'p.'"

He imitated the sound.

"Good. Isn't this easy?"

He slowly nodded, as if afraid to commit.

"Now, 'b,' Ben. Like the sound at the beginning of your name, 'b'"; I accentuated my mouth. "What does your mouth do when you make that sound? Do it again."

He repeated the sound.

"Does your mouth stay closed?"

"No."

"That's right, it's open at the end. Try it again."

"'B.'" He was more aware of his mouth.

I handed him the mirror. "See, Ben? What is your mouth doing?"

He stared at me.

"Is it open or closed?"

"It's open."

"Yes, and it's popping, too. Watch again." I repeated the "b" sound.

He smiled and made "b" sounds in front of the mirror.

"Great. Now let's look at the 'p' and 'b' sounds. Does your mouth stay in the same shape for both?"

Ben made both sounds. "Yes."

"Good. It 'pops' for both. Is your tongue making the pop or your lips?"

Ben thought and was silent.

"Make the sounds again."

He did. "My lips."

"That's right! So we call the 'p' and 'b' sounds 'Lip Poppers.'" I pointed to the picture on the desk. "See the lips and the small cloud of air coming out? Hold your hand up to your mouth." Ben did that. "Make the sound 'p' and feel the air coming out."

Ben smiled.

"Now let's look at the difference between the 'p' and 'b' sounds. We said our lips make the same shape, so how are they different? They sound different, don't they?"

Ben nodded, now fully engaged.

"Here, take your hand and put it up to your throat. Now make the 'p' sound."

I gently took his hand and had him cover his throat.

"Do you feel anything?"

Ben shook his head.

"Now the 'b' sound. Keep your hand around your throat."

Ben's eyes got big.

"Did you feel something?"

Ben smiled. "Yes."

"Our throats make noise on the 'b.' We call it the 'Noisy Brother' and the 'p' the 'Quiet Brother.'"

I turned away for a moment to check something in the manual and in my peripheral vision, watched as Ben kept saying the two sounds and feeling his throat. I knew something was clicking. The program had stressed self-discovery on the child's part. Not to spoon-feed them the answers, but through questioning, to help the child discover the answers for himself. Zina had called it the Socratic Method. It was easy to forget and skip ahead, to tell him the answer, and there were times when he was struggling, when I narrowed it down to a couple of choices. Yet, overall, I knew that by allowing Ben the opportunity to work through it, he would retain more and comprehend more.

I tried to mimic Zina's skill and fluidity but without success. I kept referring to the manual, and figured I couldn't hurt him if I did something out of sequence. I kept notes as Zina had suggested, and when Ben and I broke for a couple of days, it was helpful to refer to. By the end of the first week, I wrote:

June 18. Able to arrange pictures of the eight brothers and three cousins. Minimal prompting. Tried two-block tracking such as p/t and s/ch. Way too early for this and backed off.

Ben couldn't differentiate the changes in consonant sounds represented by the different colored blocks. It was too soon. The manual was an incredible help; it covered receptive and expressive exercises, error handling, and how to progress.

The next day I worked with just pictures and sounds without the letter symbols. We also read three pages in a book we'd picked out together. Slowly, but daily, he worked on the consonant combinations. He progressed to tracking sound changes, with letter symbol matching, as well as placing pictures below the sounds he heard.

What struck me was how Ben was able to grasp the sounds with the use of the sensory feelings. I watched my son hold the mirror in front of his mouth, saw his fingers come to his mouth and throat and feel what he was hearing, uttering. It was as if someone had untied his arms from his sides, and he could finally catch a ball being thrown to him. Before the ball had bounced off him, falling to the ground in front of him.

After two weeks of intensive work, Ben and I finished the consonant groupings and progressed to the vowel circle. Movements of the mouth, lip, and jaw grouped the vowels. These sounds were harder to discriminate for Ben. Short "i" and "e" were particularly difficult. Despite this, when I put my fingernail up to my mouth and showed him how much more open the short "e" sound was, and had him mimic this, he was able to click into the auditory difference.

We took it one step at a time, and I was able to build chains of nonsense words that contained both consonants and vowels. I had him touch and say the sounds from each chain. I compiled a set of index cards containing sight words and used them as flash cards. We covered the "sliders"—those vowel combinations that make the mouth slide into two positions. For example, "oi" as in "oil" and "ue" as in "use" were considered sliders. Ben would watch closely as I'd model the sounds for him and then hold a mirror to his mouth and study himself as he made the sounds. We also worked on the "crazy r's"—those combinations of vowels with the letter "r" such as "er," "or," and "ar."

For the first time in his life, Ben was able to start to attack the sounds of words and integrate the sounds together. I sat next to him as we held a book together.

"Look at the word, Ben."

"Mon . . ." He looked at me.

"Don't look at me. Look at the word."

"Monga."

I pulled out a sheet of paper and wrote phonetically what he said. With one hand I covered the word in the book and pointed to the paper. "This is what you said. Now look at the word in the book." I uncovered the word in the book. "See the difference? Slow down. Take it one sound at a time for now."

His head bent down. "'M.'"

"Right, a 'nose sound.' Good. What next?"

"'O.'"

"What's that called?"

"An open sound?"

"Right, an open vowel sound." I opened my mouth, exaggerating a short "o" sound. Just then, Peter popped out of his room with a newly created Lego sculpture.

"Look, Mama." He held it up proudly.

"Oh, my. What is it, Pete?"

"It's a helicopter-boat. See?" He put his little fingers up to the top. "These make it fly and here at the bottom," his fingers moved to the ski-like shapes below, "these make it float on the water."

"That's really neat. I'm glad you showed me. You've been playing very nicely, but I'm not quite finished with Ben. I'd like you to play some more now."

Pete's blue eyes went to Ben and then to me. My eyes must have wavered.

"I don't want to play anymore."

"Now, Peter."

"Okay . . ." He went sullenly back to his room a few feet away.

I watched him go and kept thinking that I must be utterly and completely crazy to consider another child when I was already stretched so thin. I tried to think how I could do all this and take care of an infant. Should we just forget about the adoption? I took a cleansing breath of air. No decisions needed to be made right now. "Okay, Ben. Where were we?"

"'N.' Another 'nose.'" He pointed to the word he was stuck on.

"Right. Because you can't make that sound with your nose closed. Very good."

"'K.' A quiet Tongue Scraper."

"Fantastic. What do you have so far?"

"Monk." He stared at the page. "Monkey. It's monkey." His face glowed.

"Right! A 'smile sound' vowel at the end—'ee.' That 'y' makes the 'e' say its name."

And so it went. Slow at first, but by the end of July, he was able to read beginner reader books. It was a start, a very solid start. There was much more to the LiPS program that I hadn't covered yet: tracking syllable changes, suffixes and prefixes, so many things. But there was time.

I started to see changes in Ben. Suddenly, he took an interest in books. As reward for his hard work, instead of a toy, we went to the bookstore, where he picked out his own books. Trips to the public library were fun for him. He developed an interest in history, particularly World War II.

The intellectual in me was fascinated with these teaching methods. The scholar in me couldn't quit analyzing the contrasts between technology with its speed and efficiency, and the sensory information only humans possess and can share with one another. The mother in me didn't really care, my only thought being that it had helped unlock a whole new world for my son.

IN ADDITION TO THE LiPS WORK, BEN WOULD PLAY EAROBICS Step 2 about four to five times a week. He would play each game twice, which would take about thirty minutes. It was a nice complement to the Lindamood-Bell, which was hard for Ben on many days, especially as we got into the vowels.

He could play Earobics Step 2 without me sitting beside him the whole time. It gave him a sense of independence and freedom, I think. There were five games, all designed to improve auditory development and target different skills, such as following auditory directions, auditory memory, phoneme segmentation, word closure skills, paying attention to auditory sounds, and word discrimination. The games were graphically engaging, and he could repeat the cue and also pause the game. He enjoyed the progress chart as the "marbles" filled with color and allowed him to see his gains.

Ben still struggled with following directions, especially in the game, "Calling All Engines." For example, the oral direction might be: "Click on the one *or* the nine." But this difficulty seemed to be with decoding the rules of language rather than de- coding sounds. The game, "Paint by Penguin," challenged him as the degree of difficulty in identifying the individual phonemes became more pronounced. But Ben used adaptive skills like counting when he could and repeating the instructions out loud.

There were days when he absolutely didn't want to do any- thing. I understood this and tried not to make the work in any way punitive. I would remind him of what he was able to do now that he couldn't do before and reason with him that it was due to his efforts on LiPS and Earobics. Some days, that reminder would make him compliant. Some days, I was firm, insisting that this was our job, and we needed to get ready for school in the fall. But over the hot summer weeks, I could see evidence of him coming out of his depression. He was belly-laughing again, had anima- tion in his emotions, and verbalized his feelings more. So on those days when I sensed he was tired or a bit down, I'd just let him play.

AT THE END OF JULY, ZINA OFFERED ANOTHER LINDAMOOD- Bell Learning Processes seminar on "The Nancibell Visualizing and Verbalizing for Language Comprehension and Thinking" or V/V. Unlike the LiPS program, this course lasted only two days, and John took some time off to be with the boys so I could attend.

I wasn't sure if Ben needed help with comprehension, but with his expressive needs, I figured it couldn't hurt. It seemed easier this time, as compared with the LiPS. I knew where I was going, Ben had made significant progress with his decoding and read- ing, and it was the summertime. No school. No sitter to pay. Just time to learn.

Zina welcomed me warmly, and this time around the other students included two public-school teachers from an outlying town. One, a tall, skinny woman, had a great sense of humor. Her associate, a tall, thin, thirtyish man, taught fourth grade and had

had success with teaching math using another Lindamood-Bell program. The teachers' tuition had been paid for by grant money they'd applied for—they hadn't been particularly encouraged to do this by their superiors. I was the Lone Mom and still felt identified by this role.

Zina seemed more relaxed, and I found the program fun to learn. It was based on Gestalt—seeing the whole of something—and making mental pictures.

After a few opening remarks about V/V, Zina said, "You know when you're reading late at night and you stop and think to yourself, 'I don't remember a word I just read'?"

Lots of nods from around the room.

"What happened is that pictures didn't form in our brains because we were either sleepy or distracted or not attending. Now for us, this is an occasional problem. For kids with language comprehension issues, it may be like that all the time. This program helps to teach those kids how to make mental pictures so that they can comprehend what they read."

I thought back to reading and my love of the written word. How the best books evoked strong images and strong emotions inside me. How I made mental pictures when I wrote. I was struck again at what a loss it would be for a child—a person—not to have this ability.

Zina continued to explain the techniques and how the imaging was built step by step from pictures to words to sentences to paragraphs. How the child was asked questions based on "structure words"—what, size, color, mood, and so on. The aim was to have the child verbalize what images he saw, trying to get more and more detailed information about those images.

Zina had us hold a picture in front of us, which was supplied at the end of the manual. She divided us into partners, one holding the picture and the other trying to elicit verbalizations about the picture.

I hadn't seen the picture Zina handed to my partner. But the structure words in front of me were my guide. My partner told me she saw a picture of a girl along the beach holding an umbrella.

"How big is the girl?"

"What color is the umbrella?"

"What is in the background?"

"Can you say if there is a mood to the picture? Is it happy or sad or relaxed?"

"Can you tell if there is any movement in the picture?"

When we were finished, she had described the picture she held in many, many words. I raised my hand and Zina said, "Yes?"

"There's a lot going on here, isn't there? I mean, there's imaging and expression and details and all kinds of things."

Zina's face opened and her black eyes seemed to intensify. "Oh, yeah. Lots going on. Lots of great stuff for the kids. It literally opens up a mental world to them."

I left after those two days excited about working with my son.

IT WAS ALMOST AUGUST AND THE NEW SCHOOL YEAR WAS only a few weeks away. I started to incorporate some V/V techniques in with the LiPS when I worked with Ben. After the preliminary steps, we were ready to start on the picture-to-picture step. One of the pictures in the manual seemed to suit him, the picture of a little boy sitting on some grass facing a duck. I copied the picture, colored it, and protected it with clear Con-Tact paper.

"Okay, Ben. Don't let me see the picture. Can you describe it to me?"

"Describe?"

"Tell me what you see."

"I see a boy."

"What does the boy look like?"

"He has yewwo hair."

"You mean blond hair?"

Ben touched his hair. "Blond."

"What is the boy doing?"

"Sitting."

"Is he alone?"

He looked at me, puzzled.

"What else is in the picture?"

"A bird."

"What kind of bird?"

He held the picture up a bit. "A white bird."

"Is it a duck?"

"Yeah. A duck."

And so on. He didn't volunteer any information, and it was detail by detail. At least his most recent eye examination showed his visual tracking was now where it should be. The eye muscles had been exercised enough with his increase in reading to get a good report from the pediatric optometrist. Ben was catching up on so much that he'd missed. Vocabulary. The ability to verbalize in a stream of sentences. My only fear was that school was going to start before we were ready.

A COUPLE OF DAYS BEFORE THE MONTESSORI PARENT OPEN house, I printed out some information on auditory processing disorder from the ASHA, the American Speech-Language-Hearing Association. The suggestions for the classroom dovetailed into the needs of a child with APD, such as preferential seating, rephrasing, speaking slowly, and giving time for a response. I made about five copies, knowing this year Ben would have several teachers, and dropped them off at the front office for the principal, Mrs. Boyle, to distribute. I included a cover letter asking her to do this for me prior to the night of the open house.

The four of us arrived on a balmy late summer night. Peter was excited to see Mrs. Minett and a new teacher, a young man with talents in Spanish and music.

We took the boys on the tour of the elementary school, a separate building from the preschool areas. Mrs. Boyle greeted us in the math room where she would be Ben's teacher.

She spoke quickly, "I didn't have time to review the handout you left at the front office, but rest assured I will before school starts." She turned toward Ben. "Ben, we're going to learn all kinds of things about math this year. We're going to get into multiplication. Do you know what two times two is?"

Ben looked at her with a total blank. She spoke hurriedly. I could hardly understand her. Ben's eyes wandered to the walls and floor, anywhere but her face.

"It's four. We're going to have lots of fun."

I reached for Ben's hand and gave her a fixed smile. Another parent walked in, whom she turned her attention toward, and I felt dismissed.

We walked on through the hallway and entered the reading room. I asked which teacher would be working with Ben. A woman with long graying hair gave me a half smile.

I said, "Ben has some difficulty with his hearing." I'd learned that this was one of the easiest ways to describe APD. "It's in the way he processes sounds. Have you ever heard of auditory processing disorder?"

"No." She looked totally confused.

I felt like a sixty-second sound bite on APD. A damn commercial. I continued, speaking too fast, falling into my words. Then, I did the same thing with the science teacher, the social studies teacher, and the music teacher. I felt sick to my stomach and the unair-conditioned school smelled stuffy and close.

John and I agreed to separate. I would join Mrs. Boyle and the other parents in the gym for her opening school year remarks while he watched the boys outside on the playground.

The gym was hotter and stuffier than the main building. Tired-looking parents crowded into the bleachers. Mrs. Boyle talked about the Indiana standardized testing, and the testing done at the Montessori school. The Montessori school kids' scores were far above the public-school children. I looked around, nodding at familiar faces. I started to fan myself with one of Mrs. Boyle's handouts. The security of the known welcomed me, and my anger subsided.

Then Mrs. Boyle started to talk about homework and book reports. Tonight, she said, each of us parents would receive a scroll of paper to construct a time line with our children. I felt sick again, as if I didn't belong here. The other parents didn't need to do commercials on their children's special learning needs.

Out of the corner of my eye, I saw John standing in the door-way of the gym. He kept looking back to the playground, I assumed to make sure the boys were okay. I sat up and saw his stiff posture, his drawn face where there was usually the hint of a grin. His eyes aggressively sought out mine.

I got up, despite Mrs. Boyle's continued oration. I clanked down the bleachers as quietly as I could and reached John's side. "What's wrong?"

"We're leaving. Now."

"Why? What's going on?"

I followed him outside where John firmly called for the boys to get off the climbing bars and swings. Ben's hair looked wet on one side.

I kept silent until we were almost to the car, deciding John wasn't going to answer me until he was ready. "Well?" I asked as we entered the car.

"A kid spit on Ben."

I turned toward Ben, whose eyes seemed sad and resigned. "Why?"

"Hell if I know." John wrestled to get the car keys out of his pocket and started the engine. "I asked Ben if it'd happened before and he said, 'yes.'"

I swallowed, confused.

"He's not going back, Karen. I'm not paying for my kid to be spit on. This isn't the place for him."

"Not going back," I whispered. "But the public school has been in session for eight days. He's missed over a week of school there. We made our decision."

"We can make a new one. He'll catch up on the work he's missed."

John allowed me a lot of freedom, and I cherished that. But I knew when he'd made up his mind about a matter, and I also knew deep, deep inside me that he was right. My body felt rigid despite the heat. "But—"

"The kid just spit on him and made a game out of it. I told him to stop, and he just laughed. I'm not sending Ben back there."

"What about Peter?"

"We'll decide that later."

"Ben, do you get spit on a lot?" The words were awkward.

"Sometimes."

"Do you like that school?"

He shrugged his shoulders in the darkness. "It's okay."

The ride home was silent for a while, and my thoughts blurred together, like the rope in a game of tug-of-war had suddenly been heaved to one side and then just as suddenly to the other side. My mind went back to last November when I met Mrs. Perkins at the public school. Her kindness. Her simplicity.

"He'd get some speech services at the public school." My voice was low and heavy.

John murmured something. His hands tightened around the steering wheel. He didn't often get mad, but when he did it was real and intense.

We arrived home, and all four of us carried the tension from the car into the house. After Peter's bath, we sent him to bed. We took Ben aside and tried to explain he wasn't going back to the school he'd known for two years. There were many reasons, but they all came to the same conclusion: It wasn't a good fit for our son anymore.

Ben cried, but it wasn't the severe reaction I'd anticipated. We tried to explain that the friends he'd make at the new school would be closer to where he lived. He'd only be ten minutes from home. The more we talked, the worse his anxiety became, so we finally quit trying to explain.

After another hour or so, we all settled down to bed. As my head touched the pillow, the tick-tock ominously stopped. The alarm rang in my head. And I felt a strange relief. I didn't know what the new school would bring, but I hadn't realized until that night how much responsibility I felt toward Ben. Obsessive Mom. Fearful Mom. And along with that feeling was a deeper feeling of being inadequate. I wasn't trained in speech and language issues. I wasn't a specialist in auditory processing. All I knew was that there wasn't much out there to help my son, and I'd done the best I could. I just prayed it'd been enough.

DURING THAT LONG NIGHT, MY MIND STARTED TO REVIEW the past few months and a huge decision John and I had made. In the spring, we'd visited a private adoption agency in Indianapolis to discuss our options about adding a baby girl to our family. After reviewing a videotape that discussed how adoption worked, the legal risks in adoption, the various types of adoption—including open and foreign adoptions—the head of the agency spoke with us. She was an adoptive mom herself and had been frank and forthcoming: Our ages would greatly limit our chances of successfully adopting a baby domestically. Our preference for a girl would also hinder the process. Most birth mothers would want a couple that was younger with no previous children. And we didn't want an open-adoption situation.

International adoption seemed the best way for us to go. She mentioned a few agencies in Indiana that handled foreign adoptions. But I'd found an agency in Tulsa, Oklahoma—of all places—that had impressed me. They were one of the few agencies that had included a list of recent clients with their literature. The three women I'd contacted sang high praises for the agency, their ethics, and how the agency had helped them every step of the way. The process was daunting. So much paperwork. So many of the steps that were out of one's control.

The agency handled adoptions through Russia, China, South America, and India. I'd never heard of foreign adoptions through India before, and I found out that the Indian government wouldn't allow pictures of their babies posted on the Internet. India did, however, allow for their babies to be escorted to the country. With John's hectic job, and not having anyone to watch Ben and Pete if we traveled, escorting seemed like a wonderful solution. The Indian babies were given up by their birth mothers due to economic hardship. And they came home at a fairly young age—prior to nine months, usually. The agency had a close relationship to the orphanage in Calcutta, and the orphanage director had made many trips to the United States to bring babies to their adoptive families.

John and I agreed India seemed our best choice. It felt right. As if designed in the cosmos, this American woman, born and raised in the Midwest, was meant to mother a little baby from around the world. It seemed as though the gap in my heart was filled with each step of paperwork we'd completed. First there was the application to the agency, the Immigration and Naturalization documents, including fingerprints of both John and me, letters of recommendation from friends, then the home study, where a social worker made two trips to the house and spoke with Ben and Peter about the adoption. She checked the house for safety, not necessarily spotlessness, thank God, and had separate interviews with both John and me.

Each step took days, weeks, or even months. The bank had approved our adoption loan in April. We'd made our pre-application to the agency July 1. As soon as our home study was accepted by the agency, the next step was getting a referral of a specific child— our daughter. But after the scene at the Montessori school earlier that night, I wondered about canceling our plans.

Although the covers rested on me, I felt exposed and cold. A deep, intensive fear took hold of me. What had I done? How could I provide for Ben's needs with a baby? Peter would be all the more shorted of my time and attention. Yet when I thought of another child, a baby, an almost joyous feeling filled me. I'd told John it was the biggest leap of faith I'd ever taken.

My friendship with Rosa had ended. Small things reflected bigger differences. I thought she was being critical when she commented about the "junk food" on my kitchen counter; she thought she was being helpful. But tonight, I longed to share some of my feelings with her, to have her make me laugh. All the confusion made me feel claustrophobic, like I needed air.

"John, are you asleep?" I asked as he snored.

"What?"

"Wake up."

"What?"

"Are we doing the right thing? I mean, about adopting?"

"Yes."

"Wake up."

"Okay."

"Maybe if you sit up."

John managed to sit up. "What's the matter?"

"I can't sleep. I'm worried about Ben and now this new baby that's coming."

Silence.

"What if I can't do it?"

"You can." He rubbed his eyes. His big hands reminded me of a bear being roused out of hibernation.

"Maybe we should tell the adoption agency that we can't do it."

"No! I want this child. We're going to get a daughter."

I needed to hear the sureness of his words. I needed to know that he wanted this child as much as I did. "Did we do the right thing, taking Ben out of school?"

John's voice lost all its sleepy slur. "Yes."

"Will he be okay? Have we done enough?"

"Sure. He's come a long way. He's scared, which is normal. I think he'll do fine in the public school. He can get speech and more help."

"What about the baby? I worry I can't do it, John. I'll be forty in December. I should have kids in middle school." I chuckled shallowly.

John nodded. "We'll do it together. I want this child as much as you. I think it'll be good for Ben and Pete." He gently smoothed the hair back from my forehead. "Studies have shown that the more siblings there are in the right families, the better the life outcome for the children."

I wondered just what journal he was quoting from, but somehow it made sense. With two male children, the comparisons with Ben and Peter had always happened, even without conscious thought. Now, with a third child, there would be more balance. And Obsessive Mom wouldn't be allowed anymore. There just wouldn't be enough time.

I tried to defog my brain with all the conflicting thoughts. "I forgot to ask. How was your day? You mentioned that one patient was pretty violent."

"Yeah. He threatened again to kill me if I didn't give him the pain meds he wanted." John slumped again into his pillow.

"Could he hurt you?"

"Sure. He's been in the military. A huge guy. But I'm careful and have security go with me." He rubbed his face again. "It's sad. There's no place for these people to go and get long-term treatment. For the poor, those options just don't exist anymore."

"I'm sorry, John. Go back to sleep."

"It'll be okay." John kissed me and turned over. He had taught himself when in his residency to fall asleep immediately. He had this ability to close his eyes and drift off. Soon I heard his smooth breathing.

"Thanks, John. I love you."

I turned over and listened to the air conditioner grinding outside my window. I thought of the boat and how the water was almost blue, but I'd realized that the lavender color had a beauty of its own. And I was thankful it was so close to blue. We were adrift, circling an island, wondering and fearful of what we'd find next. We would know soon with Ben's entrance into a new school and the arrival of our daughter. Had I helped Ben to learn enough despite his purple water? Was I trying to capture something I'd lost that was better left forgotten? Even as I felt John's warm presence next to me in bed, I worried that the weight of another child would capsize us all.

CHAPTER FOURTEEN

Entering the System

THE NEXT MORNING, PETER WENT TO JOANNE'S, THE SITTER I'd used since Ben was at the university clinic, and I was again thankful for this woman's open heart and flexibility. John and I drove Ben to the orange brick, one-story elementary school. My mouth felt dry, and I kept sliding Ben glances to make sure he was okay. I couldn't protect this child of mine, this seven-year-old boy, by myself anymore. He was in an academic and social world of his own, and I needed help. I'd thought of home-schooling many times, but John and I agreed he needed interaction with others, to be fed as much orally and aurally as possible. However, I hadn't ruled out the possibility entirely.

I'd read in the local newspaper that the school corporation had hired a new principal, someone from the Indianapolis area, a Dr. Irwin. I knew nothing about her. John held Ben's hand tightly as we entered the school. Ben's anxiety level was off the charts. Nothing we did or said made any difference, and we tried everything from encouragement to firmness. We reminded him that this was our decision as his parents, not his, when he begged to stay at the Montessori school. I felt like I had somehow betrayed him, reneged on a promise. I wondered if I could hold myself together and not make a fool of myself. John was as steady as ever, even calm.

The lobby of the school, although not air conditioned, seemed cooler than the hot morning air outside. We stepped into the administrative offices where the secretary hung up the phone and greeted us with a bright smile. I recognized her from last November.

I'd called Bridget, my local friend, the night before, and she told me to bring Ben's social security card, his birth certificate, and his immunization record to enroll him in public school. I'd fished the documents out last night and now had them ready to hand to the secretary. I explained we wanted to enroll our son, Ben, and that we probably needed to talk to the principal. After handing me a packet of forms, the secretary went briefly into a side office and came out, telling us that Dr. Irwin was available. We were ushered into a simple office with a big window behind a desk. It was 7:30 A.M. Twelve hours ago, Ben was at the Montessori School's Open House.

A petite attractive woman with curious eyes and light auburn hair styled in a blunt, curly haircut faced us. She looked like she was in her early fifties, and there was intelligence and a reserve in her movements as she stood and shook our hands. While her demeanor wasn't off-putting, it led me to think she could handle almost any situation.

After I introduced the three of us, I said, "My son will need to be enrolled in second grade. He's completed first grade at the Montessori school down the road."

I waited while she nodded an acknowledgment.

"He has an auditory processing disorder." I looked briefly at Ben, knowing his stress level was so high, he probably wasn't listening to what any of us was saying. "Are you familiar with that?"

"No. But why don't you explain it to me."

I went into my two-minute commercial and squeezed Ben's arm. Physical contact with him helped me as much as him. I also told her about some of John's history and encouraged him to speak to that, which he did.

"We just feel that with his need for speech services, and the need to be closer to his friends, that this is the better school for him now." I hesitated. "And something happened last night that concerned us." I briefly explained the event.

Dr. Irwin's eyes narrowed, and she clearly seemed repulsed by what had happened. "Ben, what's your favorite thing about school?"

"Math," he barely whispered, looking up at the ceiling and around the walls.

"He's really good at math," I added.

"Well, math is really, really important," Dr. Irwin replied. "You know, Ben, this is my first year, too. Maybe we can learn together."

Ben's eyes stopped moving around the ceiling, and he stared at her while she spoke.

She continued, "We'll know that we started together. We'll count the years together."

Her voice was so calm and reassuring. I leaned forward. "You won't do any testing on him right now, will you?"

"No," she said softening, glancing at me, and then John. "I wouldn't do that to you. In fact, my sister's child has some difficulties, and I advised her to wait a bit for tests as well. I mean, they can be very helpful. But we can decide all that later. Let's give Ben a chance to get used to us."

My body relaxed, and the visions of a hot white light staring into Ben's face as shadowy psycho-educational testers in the background yelled off questions to him vanished. I knew the image was crazy. I knew it wasn't like that. I also knew with Ben's language and auditory difficulties, it would take a very skilled person to accurately assess his real abilities.

"Okay. Let me look at the current enrollment. We have two classes per grade, so I'll need to assign him to one. . . ." She opened a drawer and studied a sheet of paper.

I took a quick inventory of Ben. Still stiff and scared, changing his position frequently. John looked antsy and kept looking at his watch. Just then his pager sounded, and I realized how I hated that damn thing. He excused himself to look for a phone.

Dr. Irwin murmured. "It looks like Mrs. Perkins has the fewest students."

"How many is that?"

"Twenty-six."

"For one teacher?"

"She also has a teacher's assistant."

God, it seemed like a lot of kids in one room, but I said, "I met her last fall, actually. We were considering a move back then, but decided to give the other school another year. She welcomed me, inviting me inside her room, and explained how things were done. I mean," I let out a weak chuckle, "she didn't know me from Adam and was very kind."

John walked back into the room and smiled reassuringly at Ben and me. "Do you have to go?" I asked, thinking there might be an urgent situation at the hospital.

"No. Just the unit calling with a question."

Dr. Irwin said, "We'll schedule a conference with you in the next week to ten days. We'll be in touch, and I'm sure we'll have Mrs. Perkins there and probably our speech therapist. We'll need you to fill out the emergency notification card and pay for his lunch if you want him to eat in the cafeteria. You can take the rest of the forms home."

I nodded. 8:05 A.M.

Dr. Irwin stood up. "Well, Ben, let's go down and meet Mrs. Perkins."

"Should we go with him?" I asked.

"Just a little way. Then you can say good-bye."

Before leaving the administrative suite, we told the secretary we'd be picking him up and bringing him to school—he wouldn't be riding the bus. Then the four of us walked down the hallway a short way. Dr. Irwin stopped, and I gave Ben a hug. "Everything is fine. You're okay. Mommy will pick you up at three o'clock."

He looked at me, helpless, and swallowed. He was definitely not okay.

Dr. Irwin gently guided him down the hallway while John and I watched him enter a room.

John and I exited the building. Ben was now enrolled in a new school with a new teacher. My plans for the year had changed completely in less than twenty-four hours. I started to cry, embarrassed, and quickly entered the car. John held me for a while. Then I broke away, saying, "It's really up to Ben now, isn't it?"

A FEW DAYS LATER, ANOTHER MOTHER TOLD ME HOW BEN had clung to the chain link fence around the playground, asking when I was coming to pick him up. Memories from three years ago and the preschool playground came to me. Yet I knew the child others were seeing wasn't the Ben I knew today. He had more expressive skills. He had better self-awareness and infinitely more receptive skills. I just didn't know how long it would take him to open up and start trusting.

We'd decided to keep Peter at the Montessori school. John and I had talked about what was best for each son. One person had told me her decision to place her three sons was based on "each son's needs each year." Peter was thriving under Mrs. Minett's care. Didn't I owe the same consideration to Peter that I gave to Ben—what was best for him? And the Montessori school was a fine school. I'd leveled with Nancy, the administrator at the school, about our reasons for withdrawing Ben. It just wasn't a good fit for Ben anymore. They'd been gracious, assuring us that Ben could return at any time.

It was the end of Ben's first week at the public school. I got into the car and drove to pick him up, my leg muscles stiff from tension. I waited in line for a few minutes before moving my van up in the school dismissal line, and Mrs. Perkins opened the door. She must have read the worried look on my face. "He's fine. He's had a good day."

Ben climbed into the car and I murmured, "Thanks," as she shut the side door.

"Okay, how was your day?"

"I want to go back to the other school. I miss Monty. I promise to be good." His eyes filled up with tears. Since Frank had changed schools last year, Monty had become one of his few friends. I felt bad that he hadn't had a chance to say good-bye to him.

"Honey, it has nothing to do with you. You aren't being punished. This school is better for you this year."

"Where Peeda go?" His mood had changed to sullen.

"Peter is going to stay at the Montessori school. He's not old enough to go to this school yet."

Silence.

"Let's just go home."

Silence.

MRS. PERKINS AND DR. IRWIN WERE TRUE TO THEIR WORD, CALLING me within a week to set up a meeting. The speech therapist, Amy, was also there. A woman in her forties, she was responsible for the speech services of several of the local schools and only came to this elementary building on a part-time basis. Her short frosted hair framed a pretty, open face, and the softness of her spoken words almost matched Mrs. Perkins's voice.

Mrs. Perkins sat slightly hunched over a stack of papers. Dr. Irwin had a pen and pad handy and started by asking, "How do you think Ben is doing?"

"I know the change came without any warning or lead time for him to make the slightest adjustment mentally. He was thrust into a new school with new kids and new teachers. I think he's still anxious, but I think he'll relax eventually. I hope he's given that time." I looked at Amy, thinking about the speech and language tests that were bound to come.

Mrs. Perkins spoke up. "Well, I have to be honest with you." She looked directly at me with clear blue eyes. "If the kids were in a pack all together, Ben isn't even at the back. He's trailing way behind."

I took a breath and held it.

She shuffled some papers. "These are from last Friday. Three days ago." She pushed them toward me. Blanks, empty lines, incorrect responses.

After briefly studying the papers, I said, "I know he knows some of this stuff."

Mrs. Perkins nodded. "Now, today, his work shows improvement. He was able to finish his work and much of it is correct."

"Well, I'm glad we didn't meet on Friday." I laughed anxiously, glad that Dr. Irwin joined me.

"I can't be there helping him all the time. I have twenty-five other kids who need me to teach them."

"I understand."

"He needs to work more independently." She folded her hands over Ben's work.

Amy turned a stapled group of papers toward me. "These are your rights as a parent regarding Ben's IEP, his Individual Education Program. He'll receive special services through speech, a Communication Disorder." She gently slid them across the table. "These are for you to keep." She went on to explain about IEPs and about my involvement in preparing Ben's program, that today, we were just starting the forms, and would meet again to formalize his plan after Ben's testing was complete.

"You'll be testing his speech and language abilities, right?"

"Yes."

"I would respectfully request that you take your time with those tests. I'll be honest with you: Ben doesn't do well on tests, and the results will be more valid if they're administered when Ben isn't anxious."

"I think you're right. I have noticed the couple of times I've seen him, he's very preoccupied with what he may be missing in class." She wrote something on her pad.

"Is there an audiologist on staff?"

"No. The school corporation contracts with one who sees children by referrals," Amy explained.

I looked down at the table. It didn't seem like enough. With all the kids who struggled with reading and learning differences—I hated the word "disabilities"—it just didn't seem like enough.

Mrs. Perkins spoke up. "I have to apologize to you. I didn't have a chance to read the handout on APD that you brought in on his first day until that afternoon. But he was given a desk at the front of the classroom and away from distracting noises in the hall by the end of the first day."

"That's great. I mean, that you had this new student and were able to move him so quickly."

Amy took the lid off her pen. "So do we want to add that to his IEP?"

Mrs. Perkins nodded. "Preferential seating. I think extra time on standardized state testing, in a smaller classroom, would be helpful for him. Speaking slowly—"

"And rephrasing. He also does better when something is explained to him using different words," I added.

Amy listened closely. "Maybe some vocabulary work, then," and jotted a notation.

We continued to discuss that Ben would receive the curriculum with accommodations, not modifications. A very important distinction, as modifications would mean deviation from his age-level curriculum. It was recommended he be placed in Reading Lab tutoring, offered daily to help with language arts. I was assured that when Ben was pulled, he would not miss any new curriculum work.

Amy, who was leading the discussion on the IEP, came to the next section on the form and said, "Here is where we list some of Ben's strengths. What do you see as Ben's strengths?" She looked at both Mrs. Perkins and me.

"He works so hard. He'll do anything I ask him to do, bless his heart," Mrs. Perkins said. She again looked straight at me. "He really tries to do his best. He wants to please so much." She paused and leaned toward all of us sitting around the table. "You know, he actually thanked me the other day. Can you imagine? A student actually thanked me."

"Polite." Amy wrote.

"Honest. With Ben, what you see is what you get," Mrs. Perkins added. "I mean, with some of the other kids, they're—I don't know—a little devious sometimes. Ben's a sweetheart."

"He is a very gentle little boy. He always has been. I know with time, he'll start to relax." I glanced around at the other faces and hoped I conveyed my belief in Ben.

Mrs. Perkins jotted something on a small Post-It note and slid it over to me. "Call me any time. This is my home phone number. I'm usually home by four-thirty, and Saturday mornings are good. Don't wait. If something is bothering you, give me a call."

We continued to talk about Ben's transition and finished the meeting a few minutes later. I'd been listened to. My input had credibility. Mrs. Perkins and Amy genuinely wanted to help my son. I felt very fortunate.

I DIDN'T FEEL LIKE GOING BACK TO THE SCHOOL, BUT I HAD no excuse not to. John was home fairly early from work, and it was still daylight, an early fall day in October, just before the leaves start to change and the last warm days linger. I thought about my daughter constantly. Had she been born yet? How was she doing? Was she held and loved enough? When would she come home? My thoughts ended as I pulled up to the elementary school parking lot and saw a few other cars parked outside the spaces usually reserved for the buses. It was my second meeting of the PTO, Parent Teacher Organization. The first one was informative, but I felt lost as to who was who, and what was what. Words like Spring Fling, Fall Festival, and Santa Shop left me a little confused. I had seen Mrs. Perkins at the last one and knew that most of the teachers did their duty and came.

My thoughts drifted back over the last few weeks. Ben seemed to be much more relaxed when we dropped him off. Mrs. Perkins sent home graded papers on Friday. Each weekend, either Jamie or I would go over the papers with Ben while he made corrections—a nice habit picked up from the Montessori school. I had a better idea of what he needed reinforcement in, and it helped him as the curriculum continued. Reading and writing were still a struggle for him, but Mrs. Perkins knew this and was working hard on it with him.

I walked into the music room, the designated room for the PTO meetings, and saw the officers sitting at a table that faced three rows of folding chairs. The room was about half full, mostly with teachers. I took inventory and saw that a dozen parents were present. Out of a student body of around 300, it was a pathetic turnout of parental support. No wonder teachers felt a disconnection from parents. I scanned the room. Most of the faces had been at the previous meeting with only a couple of new parents, including one father.

Mrs. Perkins waved brightly at me. I learned this was one of her trademark habits. There was something so genuinely warm and caring in how she used her whole arm that I couldn't help but wave warmly back at her.

The treasurer reported about the profits from the Fall Festival, which included a chili supper. I'd helped dish out desserts, vowing to think really hard about what I volunteered for in the future. The Santa Shop, I learned, was a "store" in the PTO room where children could buy gifts for their family. Envelopes were sent home and parents could put money into the envelope and list those family members the child was to buy for. The cost of each item ranged from one to five dollars.

A ripple of laughter roused me from drifting off into other thoughts. There was a rapport between the parents in attendance and the teachers, an implicit trust that the PTO was there to support the teachers as a whole. Funding of field trips was discussed and each teacher was allowed an extra field trip per year to be funded by the PTO.

It struck me how poor the county was. The contrast between

the Montessori school and the public school hit me. Parents flocked to each event at the private school, averaging 90% and better attendance rates. Here, 10% of the parents were in attendance. Yet I knew that blaming those who worked or had other responsibilities wasn't my place. Still, it seemed sad, and I crossed my arms, glad that I had come.

After some discussion of when to schedule the next meeting around Thanksgiving break, the meeting adjourned. Mrs. Perkins quickly approached me as I stood up.

"You know what?"

I shook my head.

"I figured out what Ben needs this year."

I licked my lips, wondering what she was thinking. Medicine for attention problems? More in-depth testing? A modified curriculum?

"He needs this." She began gently stroking my lower arm. "He needs nurturing and caring."

I nodded, thankful that this woman was with him when I wasn't. "How's he doing?"

She hesitated, as if she were choosing her words carefully. "He's starting to relax. He has friends. One of his favorite games is tag at recess." She slowly let her hand drop from my arm. "He just needs to know it's okay."

My eyes grew misty.

"Now, I don't baby him," she said firmly. "He's got to work hard and he does. But I don't change my expectations of him." She tilted her chin out just a little.

"That's good. That's the way I want it."

People brushed past us as they left, and I started to move with the crowd.

"Do you have a little more time?" Mrs. Perkins sat down in a vacant chair and waited until I sat beside her.

She smiled at someone passing and said in a lower, softer voice, "I know where you're coming from. My two daughters had some learning problems. Back then, all the doctor would say was that they'd grow out of it." She looked at me again, with those expressive eyes. "Well, they didn't grow out of it, and it was hard. I know how tough it is. I've been there."

I listened silently.

"I probably waited too long. But back then, they didn't have the labels they do today—although I know some labels aren't good. They didn't tell you anything." She shrugged her shoulders in a tired way. "I did what I could."

We sat there for a little while more, and I felt grateful to this woman for confiding in me, for trusting my judgment about my son, and for her humanness.

DURING THE WEEKS THAT LED UP TO THANKSGIVING, THE family fell into a new routine, with Ben in the local school and Peter at the Montessori preschool. But like one of those small plastic balls that once set in motion bounces unpredictably and wildly around, so my feelings about the adoption were mixed and contradictory. I desperately wanted this child, but was more unsure than ever that I could handle it all.

On November 29, we received the referral pictures of Anusree or Annie, as we would call her, a beautiful baby with golden tanned skin. In one picture, her eyes were closed, and she was lying on her side. There were two others, both with her facing the camera. In one, she was sucking her thumb and seemed so alone. After turning and inspecting the photos for hours, I went to the Kodak Magic Picture machine at the local drugstore and made a bazillion copies. I started to write Annie letters and found they helped me to sort out all these feelings.

Dear Annie,

I called Ruth from the adoption agency a few days ago to ask if she remembered you from her recent trip to India. She was so kind. She has a rich, soothing, loving voice and told me that she did remember you and said you seemed healthy. I asked if your biological mother would know that you would be adopted abroad and Ruth said, "No. There is much fear of family names getting out." Your birth mother would probably have left you to the care of the orphanage director. I felt sad when I hung up. I felt sad to get so little information. I felt sad for your biological mother and for her future yearnings for you.

We have finished all the paperwork and our home study was accepted last month. The dossier is in India being processed by the courts. Three long months to wait wondering how you are, if you are loved enough, ever cry for too long.

Many times I have wondered where this path will lead you and me. All I know is that there has been this guidance from Him. Once I thought about adoption, it never has let me go. I am a bit frightened, not knowing how I will handle three. John's hours are long, but if it wasn't for his devotion to his children, I couldn't do this. He is a wonderful man, your father. An honest, decent man who has had a hard life in many ways.

I hope you come to us soon because I also know that you have already made me happy. Love, Mom.

CHAPTER FIFTEEN

Liberty

THE CHRISTMAS BREAK FINALLY CAME, AND BEN NEEDED THE respite. Although school tired him, and when he came home he was hungry and fatigued, there were no signs of the depression he'd experienced in first grade. Luckily the only homework that Mrs. Perkins requested was to have the child read at least ten minutes each night and review his spelling words for the Wednesday test. John faithfully sat down with Ben every night to read. After Ben would finish, he chose a book for Dad to read to him.

Ben had also joined Cub Scouts in the fall on the recommendation of Mrs. Perkins, and he'd enjoyed seeing friends outside of school. I liked the Cub Scout Motto ("Do your best"), and the Cub Scout Promise was one of the first texts that Ben was able to recite from memory.

Mrs. Perkins would call me periodically to tell me about a particular area that Ben was struggling with, such as "greater than/less than" and telling time. Those calls made a tremendous difference. I could reinforce the concepts being presented in class and avoid Ben feeling that he was being left behind. Mrs. Perkins's tone was never impatient, just matter-of-fact: This is what Ben needs extra help with.

Since Annie was due to come home sometime in March or April, we decided that we should visit the Southwest and John's family over the holidays while we just had the two boys. This time we planned to fly into Phoenix where his parents had their winter home.

The airline upgraded us to first class when our original flight was overbooked. Peter sat next to John, looking out his window. Suddenly, he turned and said, "God lives up here, right?"

John nodded.

The billowy clouds' water crystals sparkled like glitter as the sun shone from above.

Peter kept peering and straining out the window and finally announced. "I don't see him."

John assured him God was there, however.

"You know, Ed told me there was no Santa Claus." Ed was a little friend of Peter's at school.

I heard John's voice say, "Is that right?"

Peter laughed. "Yeah. Do you know who he says is really Santa?"

"No."

"This is really funny. Ed thinks it's the parents. And he's so silly because first," Peter put a finger in the air, "that would cost a lot of money to buy all those presents and that's a lot of money for parents to have."

"That's true."

"And second. This is the biggest reason." Another finger in the air. "Where would parents get the elves?"

He went on to state that he'd never seen elves around parents. Santa had elves. Proof, by Peter's reasoning, that Santa did exist.

Peter, apparently satisfied with his logic, began playing with the tray table on the back of the seat in front of him until John asked him to stop.

Ben thought the take-offs and landings were thrilling, like riding a fair ride. His relaxed face helped to soothe my fears as the plane bumped along with normal air turbulence.

Perhaps because I'd lived in landlocked, relatively flat land all my life, I found mountain ranges fascinating. The Superstition Mountains near Phoenix held my attention each time I saw them in the distance while riding in my father-in-law's car. John's father took us to the foothills to look for Apache Tears or obsidian. He knew that rock hunting and the study of natural minerals had become a hobby of John's. The boys stayed with their grandfather in the lower area where we'd parked the car, while John and I hiked up a short distance. I puffed and panted, but it felt so good to fill my lungs and mind with nothing except the awareness of my body.

John took my hand and helped me up the last of the distance to the top. The side of the mountain had been chipped away by the thousands of people looking for the pearls of volcanic glass, or obsidian, that was buried in the fine glistening rock. Jagged edges marked the hillside that hid its secrets well.

Now I turned to look at the other side of the path and stopped. A small canyon, surrounded on three sides by layers of apricot, gold, brown, and yellow rock, stretched below me. The dry wind blew my hair sharply into my face, and the cloudless blue sky did nothing to prevent the sun from burning my lips.

"Look, Karen," John said. "Over there, under that big over-hang."

I peered to where he pointed, hundreds of feet below us. "What is it?"

"Looks like an ancient Native American shelter. It's made out of stones."

I had no idea how old the shelter was, but I wondered who'd lived there and if they had had children. How they stood the cold at night and the rainstorms. How much food they had to eat. I thought of my beloved parents, and how grateful I was—my father had made a full recovery from his open-heart surgery and was in the best shape of his entire life.

John and I stood there, together, silently. He pulled me close to him, and I hadn't felt that safe in a long time. I had a vision of a camera pulling away from the two of us into the sky, atmosphere, and into space, viewing the earth from thousands of miles away. And I thought how my life was a speck, a fleeting wink in the grand scheme of things. And somehow it brought me a great peace.

On Christmas Eve, we flew home in time for Santa and his elves to visit. As a child, I could never figure out why my mother got so cranky when we'd return from a vacation. Now, I knew. Double-digit loads of laundry faced me. Bags of mail to sort through. Bills to pay. But my sons had been able to see a real desert and experience a real cactus, and learned that oranges, lemons, and grapefruit came from trees, not the grocery store.

SECOND QUARTER REPORT CARDS WERE TO BE DELIVERED IN January and another conference had been scheduled with Mrs. Perkins and Amy. I had a hard time eating on those days, fearful that some unexpected curve would be thrown my way. I knew Amy had taken a lot of time to assess Ben's speech and language needs, and I was grateful for that.

Mrs. Perkins had been upfront and honest from the day I met her. She was the one who confided that Ben was so behind at the first of the year. Then she eased my mind at the PTO meeting and with her calls throughout the semester. Even as nervous as these meetings made me, I felt a certain trust in these people who shared my son with me.

I walked into the administrative suites, nodded to Dr. Irwin as I passed her office and was told the meeting would be in the conference room in the back. I was the first there and situated myself, arranging Ben's file that held his APD handout, copies of his report card, a copy of all the therapies and services he'd received in his young life, samples of schoolwork he'd done, especially spelling tests, and miscellaneous notes.

I looked at the clock on the wall and thought about those single parents who worked and had children who struggled. Or the parents who didn't have the time and resources to learn new techniques to help their children read and process sounds. They would have no choice but to rely on the system to help them. I shook my head and wondered how a country as rich in resources as ours couldn't offer more. There were millions of children and their parents who were suffering. I felt sad and angry. Guilty for the resources I had, and at the same time, grateful I had them.

Just then, Amy and Mrs. Perkins came in chatting with each other. Amy pulled out another copy of "Notice of Parent Rights" regarding Ben's IEP, and I waited for Mrs. Perkins to begin. Somehow, I knew today was her show.

"Mrs. Thompson, I want you to know that your son is like a sponge right now. He's just soaking it all in. We have to ask him to let other children have a turn in reading. He'll raise his hand almost every time, and we have to say, 'Ben, give someone else a chance.' I can see so many changes in him. He's really blossomed this year."

She handed me a paper. "Here's my summary of the quarter. He's so different from the little boy who came to me this August."

I took the typed page in my hand and began to read out loud: "Ben has made significant progress in all academic areas. In reading, we are at the beginning of second-grade material. Ben is confident in reading group. He knows the vocabulary and is able to discuss the story. In reading, Ben had the best score in his group on working independently at his desk. Spelling scores are excellent this quarter. Ben is so proud of his spelling and delights that he is often one of the few children who score a hundred percent on the test."

I briefly looked up and saw Mrs. Perkins and Amy grinning. I continued, "On daily work and tests, Ben's eighty-nine percent in language/English is commendable. His progress is just great! Ben is having some trouble writing a paragraph with complete sentences. This will come. We are just not there yet! Ben still has areas that are hard for him, but as you can see, his scores are well within the average range for a second-grade student. Ben has grown in many other ways this quarter. He is totally focused during group lessons. He raises his hand and gives appropriate answers to questions. At recess, Ben always plays with a group of children. He is accepted and has friends. Ben laughs a lot and talks with me. I think we can celebrate many achievements with Ben this quarter. I can see him growing in so many ways and becoming more confident each day."

At that moment, I felt an old pain lift from me. This kind teacher, this talented, caring woman, had helped me with Ben when I desperately needed someone to help make it enough. She'd reached out to him and balanced kindness with discipline in her simple rural classroom.

I finally muttered in a choked voice, "Thank you so much. This means so much to me." I studied another paper stapled to her narrative and saw my son's scores, which were average (84% in math; 89% in language; 92% in his reading group; and 97% in spelling). That blessed word: "average."

Amy went on to tell me about his current test results, summarizing that receptively he was in the normal range, but there was still a lot of expressive work to be done. She shared her goals for speech therapy with me and asked for input.

"Don't you think, though, that his spontaneous speech is better than those test scores reflect?" I couldn't help myself from asking.

Amy bit her lip as if in thought. "That might be."

"Anyway, it doesn't matter," I said. "Just that controlling side of me that won't let go, I guess." I chuckled to myself.

The three of us got to work on his IEP with recommendations for helping Ben with language and listening, much the same as before when we listed them in the fall. After the work was finished, I stood up and thanked them again.

"I'll always remember this day, Janice," I said to Mrs. Perkins, taking the liberty of addressing her by her first name. "I want to share something with you. One of Ben's therapists told me something once. I think Ben was about four at the time, when his delays were at their peak. And I'd said something to the effect that I thought Ben was a bright boy and had such a wonderful emotional feel for people. I remember this therapist looking at me and saying, 'Not everyone grows up to be a rocket scientist. Many people live fulfilling lives doing much different things. And are quite happy.'"

I looked at Janice, desperate not to cry. "I know this therapist, and she is a kind woman. She didn't mean it unkindly, but it cut into me. . . ."

Janice took my arm, pushed her chin slightly forward, and said in a firm voice, "Ben can be anything he wants to be. Anything at all."

BEN'S EIGHTH BIRTHDAY PARTY IN MARCH OCCURRED FIVE days after our new daughter, Annie, came home to us. I was my usual tense self, overwhelmed with a party for about a dozen second-graders that might as well have been an inauguration dinner for the President of the United States. And I was getting used to having a four-and-a-half month-old baby, wanting to do all the right things, getting used to her eating habits, her nap preferences, and her personality.

Annie was an absolutely beautiful baby, so tiny by American standards—eleven pounds, two ounces—but perfect. Delicate features, tiny hands and feet. She had fine, black hair and eyes that scrutinized me, studied me. I thought of all she'd gone through in her first weeks of life on earth. Each time I held her, I knew she was my daughter. Aside from some nutritional anemia and small motor delays, both of which were corrected with time, she was given a clean bill of health.

Peter was fascinated with his little sister, taking on the role of Big Brother like a tailor-made suit. He'd be upset if she cried, sing to her, talk to her incessantly, and laugh when she did something funny. Ben would smile at her and tell me, "Awww. She's cute." And when I'd watch him around his tiny new sister, Ben would gently hold his finger out for her to grasp and say, "Hi, Annie." He'd gently pick her up and carry her, his strong body easily holding her weight. My perfect baby was now helping his little sister to catch up.

Mrs. Perkins came to Ben's party, as did her assistant and several moms and their children. I watched the kids splash and swim in the indoor pool, trying to get used to the hot, chlorine-filled air. Bits and pieces of the adults' conversations caught my attention.

"I told him not to do that . . ."

"Tell her to call me . . ."

"I didn't know you were her daughter-in-law. Why, we're almost related!"

I decided I liked this little town, after all. It may be Nowhere U.S.A., but it was a place that turned out to be good for us.

A splash of water almost hit my leg. In the water, Ben reached his arm out, stretching as far as he could to tag another boy. His friend squealed and went after Ben, both laughing and spitting water out of their mouths. There was Pete, his swimming trunks needing to be retied, his life jacket hanging from him, rubbing his blue eyes and coming up to ask me something.

John was in the room with Annie, waiting for the kids to come and eat pizza. My worries about Annie and handling the needs of three children were still with me, but when I held her and touched her, I felt a renewed strength. Mrs. Perkins told me that Ben's progress had stayed steady, and at the end of the year, he received the "Most Improved Student Award."

FIVE YEARS HAD PASSED SINCE I STARTED THIS JOURNEY WITH my family. Five years that had tested me again and again. Some tests I'd failed, others I'd done okay with. But whatever judgment I could make on how I'd navigated the past, I knew in my heart that by some miracle, I'd turned out to be a better person. Ben had given me that gift. I'd try to make sure it lasted for a lifetime.

The boat had grown somehow, and held all five of us now. John was with us, and I realized he'd been there all along. I'd just taken his presence for granted, like my lungs expanding and heart beating without conscious thought. When the boat enlarged, a smaller set of oars had been added. Ben had taken hold of the new set and was rowing with strength and tenacity. He couldn't move the boat without our help yet—and I knew he would hit some choppy water in his life, as would Peter and Annie. John and I shared the other oars as I held Annie with my free arm. Peter was helping me with Annie, playing with her when I put her down. He seemed happier than I'd ever seen him. Together, as a family, we were ready to decide where we wanted to go next.

CHAPTER SIXTEEN

Hindsight and Help

A PARENT KNOWS IF THERE IS SOMETHING WRONG WITH THE child. A parent knows the child's spiritual, physical, social, emotional, and cognitive sides—the whole person. But when there is a problem with development, exactly what the problem is and what action to take are matters that are more elusive. The path that John and I traveled with Ben is unique. This memoir reflects one little boy's difficulties and his successes with various tools. It's not meant to be a steadfast guide for treatment of other children.

It's easy to make mistakes, missteps that become apparent when the tape of the past is rewound and the events are reviewed. But as one parent shared with me:

You know, a lot of people said, "Be sure to ask questions. Don't hesitate to get answers." Well, parents often don't know what questions there are to ask. It's not that they don't ask the right questions. It's that they don't know the questions exist.

This final chapter is meant to help you formulate your questions. A basic guide, but one that I wish I'd had five years ago. It's intended to provide some general signs that could prompt you to seek out answers from professionals and to illustrate how children with APD appear to the world. This chapter also tries to explain some of the various roles that professionals assume when evaluating your child. First presented are the "red flags" that can signal it's time for clinical input, with the qualification that if you as a parent feel something isn't right, follow your intuition.

Signals to Intervene

In early development—around 18 months and up—one of the first signs that there may be a problem with auditory processing is **delayed or gibberish type of speech,** reflecting that the sounds are not being processed normally. One parent described it as "garbage going in, and garbage coming out." Acoustic confusion such as when the child says "boggy" for "doggy" and other **articulation errors** suggest possible auditory discrimination problems. **Difficulty rhyming words** may be a clue that sounds are not being processed clearly. **Altered speech,** such as speaking more slowly, may help the child who cannot keep up with the pace of normal speech, and would give further evidence that APD may indeed be a problem.

Be aware that most audiologists will not be able to diagnose APD until the child is approximately six to seven years of age. However, the presence of these "red flags" and other evidence of a child's difficulty processing sounds should trigger a referral for therapy at a much younger age, usually around two and a half to three years of age. In addition, a full speech and language assessment, along with acuity testing of the auditory system (to rule out hearing loss) would be warranted given these early signs. (The National Institutes of Health recommend that all newborns be screened for potential hearing loss, which is separate from APD. In some states, this screening is now mandatory.)

In the preschool years, **a lack of attentiveness, inability to concentrate, difficulty in following directions, being easily distracted, and saying, "huh?" and "what?" frequently** may be indicators that sounds are not clear to the child. Many of these signs are exactly the same as attention deficit disorder (ADD), inattentive type. You may be advised to seek medication for your child based on a faulty or incomplete diagnosis. But to add to the complexity of it all, attention deficit disorder is seen very frequently with APD. The two disorders may be found together and separately.

During this time, the child is usually interacting with adults outside the home, such as preschool teachers, baby-sitters, day-care workers, and Sunday school volunteers. Their feedback may also reflect possible signs of APD as well as **sensitivity to sounds** and other stimulation. These individuals may also report that the child has **difficulty with social skills.** For example, if a child can't process the rules to a game, then the child may limit social interaction to one-on-one situations or seek out adult company.

A developmental or behavioral pediatrician and/or a child psychiatrist could help rule out other problems or assess your child for **anxiety** issues induced by the APD. An occupational therapist may evaluate fine motor skills as well as sensory integration issues. If not done previously, a full battery of audiological tests and speech and language assessments should also be performed.

Some children's difficulties surface with **language arts and pre-reading skills upon entering kindergarten,** when phonics is introduced. Adapting to this difficulty by sight-reading will buy the child some time, but only for a while. Sight-reading depends more upon visual memorization than word attack skills that other non-APD children possess. Again, inability to follow directions, awkward social interactions, and **difficulty decoding and integrating phonemes (reading problems) and reading comprehension** may be clues that the child needs to be evaluated for APD.

Grade school provides academic and **environmental challenges** to the APD child. Noisy rooms and distractions, from cafeteria and gym crowds to hallway marching, may thwart the child's progress. Teacher conferences provide feedback ranging from severe **academic difficulties** to "something is just not right." Issues surrounding areas of cognition or intellectual functioning, memory, and reading may cloud the underlying APD or be additional problems. At this time, a definite diagnosis of APD may be obtained. Educational testing can help to identify specific learning needs and may be added to the assessments mentioned above. Learning difficulties have an extremely high concurrence with APD. Other assessments, such as sensory integration difficulties, may be made based on the presentation of the child.

If the child has gone undiagnosed into the latter elementary years due to mild APD in conjunction with effective coping skills, **difficulty with lecture-type learning situations** may surface. Note-taking based upon auditory information may prove too difficult for the student. Where before there was academic success, a bright child may start to experience failure. A full battery of audiological testing for APD and educational testing provide necessary information to help support the child's academic efforts.

As implied in the "red flags" noted above, children with APD represent a very heterogeneous population. Indeed, children can display difficulties in any of the following areas:

- Receptive language
- Expressive language
- Articulation errors
- Word retrieval (finding the right word at the right time)
- Auditory memory
- Hearing in noisy backgrounds
- Reading
- Spelling (word attack and sight)
- Reading comprehension
- Social skills
- Acute sound sensitivity
- Organizational skills
- Motor planning skills (such as handwriting)
- Other problems such as anxiety and depression secondary to APD (may overlap with other disciplines)

There are several models of APD that attempt to categorize and profile individuals with APD by the clusters of deficits the child displays (and which testing reveals). Scholars have come a long way in understanding APD by the patterns of behaviors that are identified.

Roles of Professionals

Auditory processing deals with how a human being makes sense of sounds in the environment. While the actual prevalence of APD is not currently known, some estimates place APD as affecting as many as half of all children diagnosed with learning difficulties. Certainly, millions of children's learning is compromised due to APD. The need for qualified clinicians who are trained in the testing and diagnosing of APD is critical, as is the need for an increased awareness of APD in educational settings. The legitimacy of APD must be addressed in order that our children are given appropriate services. In other words, APD needs to be viewed as a life-impacting disorder that deserves serious attention.

In the real world, parents often receive an inferred diagnosis of APD from a variety of professionals (speech therapists, occupational therapists, and educational psychologists) based on a variety of tests that are specific to those professions. However, the audiologist trained in APD is the professional qualified to test for and conclude that the child is experiencing problems processing sounds, and thus make the official APD diagnosis. The current standard battery of testing for APD includes tests of electrophysiologic measures and behavioral measures done in a sound room under earphone conditions with an audiometer. Other reports such as behavioral checklists (Does the child say, "what?" and "huh?" frequently?) provide descriptive information on how the child processes sound, not information that can be used solely to reach an APD diagnosis.

The problems your child has or the "clinical presentation," determines the choice of specific tests run in the standard battery. The model of APD that is employed by the clinician will determine how test results are interpreted or the APD "labeled." The audiologist should work closely with the speech therapist when the child has speech and language issues.

Candidacy issues become paramount when seeking treatment of APD. Who will benefit from which treatment? It is a complicated question and a critical one for our children. Based upon the audiological evaluation, the professional should determine which intervention is right for your child. Be aware that practitioners may hold strong feelings regarding treatment tools. Some therapies are considered controversial because of possible untoward side effects, the lack of empirical data (research findings), intensity, and cost.

Briefly, therapy, treatments, and tools can include, but are not limited to:

- Auditory training (AT), which can take a variety of forms
- Auditorily based computer programs such as Fast ForWord Learning Programs and Earobics Step 1 and 2
- Frequency modulated (FM) amplification systems: personal FM units (which have a headset or individual desk receiver and are sometimes referred to as "FM Trainers") and sound field FM systems (a room equipped with loudspeakers) are transmitters and receivers designed to help the child receive a clear signal through background noise
- Multisensory reading programs such as the Lindamood-Bell and the Orton-Gillingham methods
- Modified listening programs such as Auditory Integration Therapy (AIT)
- A variety of interventions from the speech-language therapists and audiologists specifically suited to the child

The audiologist should be able to accomplish two goals for the parents after testing. First, a complete explanation of the test results should be given to the parents. When they leave the office, they should have a basic understanding of what was measured, how it was measured, and what was found. Second, the audiologist should clarify treatment options and recommend, based upon assessment findings, which of those options should be prioritized.

It's up to you, the parent, to question those recommendations as necessary, regarding the safety, efficacy, and research findings that led the audiologist to recommend that particular tool. Find out if the treatment suggested is a tool, designed to help the child cope with APD in a learning environment, or intended to be a remediation technique. In other words, make sure you understand the purpose and goal of the therapy, tool, or technique.

That being said, in order to treat the child as a whole entity, a multidisciplinary approach is often the best for the child. Frequently, it's very difficult for a parent to navigate the varied professionals who diagnose concurrent problems. For example, a medical doctor (pediatrician, family practitioner, etc.) may offer the diagnosis of pervasive developmental disorder, which indicates delays in all areas—communication, social, and developmental. The child psychiatrist may conclude there is a difficulty with attention deficit disorder. The occupational therapist may diagnose sensory integration dysfunction. An educational psychologist may find a nonspecific learning disability. The child ends up with an alphabet soup of diagnoses after his name: PDD, ADD, SID, and learning disability, unspecified. The diagnoses may be correct and still not include the underlying APD.

Or the diagnoses may be severely off the mark, due to the unknown presence of APD. Physical problems should also be ruled out by a complete physical examination, including a full vision screening/evaluation to make sure tracking and visual/spatial difficulties have been accounted for.

Often, it's you, the parent, who faces the daunting responsibility of making sense of the specialists' reports and integrating that information into a coherent whole. I use the metaphor of a geometric shape to try to understand this phenomenon. For example, suppose a child is evaluated by various individuals and the following are diagnosed: APD, SID, and expressive and receptive language disorder. A triangle is formed, each side carrying the individual diagnosis—a side for each relevant finding. In the center of the triangle is a circle that holds the child and his parents. Perhaps the circle is out of perfect symmetry and leans to one of the diagnoses. The parent knows that those three diagnoses leave out the whole of the child that they know. It is your job, a very difficult one, to communicate to those evaluators what you see and what you know to be true, and to actively contribute to a plan of action to help your child.

Interestingly, many times a parent better understands his or her own difficulties after the child is diagnosed with APD, as was the case with John. It is a moment of bittersweet insight for the adult to understand that a difficulty with reading, learning, and/or APD answers many questions pertaining to his or her own academic and career histories. After years of wondering, you realize that APD has little to do with intellect or "how smart" a person is. It is a complex disorder that twists and turns and unfolds uniquely with each individual.

Other Journeys

I have interviewed parents from around the world whose children have dealt with APD and have found the presentations of APD very mixed—the stories touching and, at times, heartbreaking. Service settings and providers varied from hearing clinics, university and private clinics, and schools to private tutors and military medical officers. Almost without exception, the Internet was used as a source of information about APD. The following case studies illustrate in human terms how APD can lie hidden as other problems surface in the child's development and the critical need for educating the world about APD. The stories below highlight the journeys taken by some of these parents and their children.

Jeremy

His mother spoke to me about Jeremy's journey. She is a caring, single parent of two sons.

As an infant, Jeremy was easily overstimulated, startling easily, and clothing tags bothered him as an infant. He babbled and earned the nickname "Jabbers" from his grandfather. He babbled nonstop with sounds.

Sometimes there were words in them. When he was about two, I knew he had a speech delay. I thought I saw improvement between the ages of two and four. But looking back, I just adjusted to hearing what Jeremy was saying. I adapted to him. When he was four, he entered into an early intervention program.

Jeremy's pediatrician wasn't concerned. He told me it was just Jeremy's age. When I started him in the early intervention program, they told me the same thing: that my son wasn't severe enough to warrant any intervention. At this point, he was talking in two- and three-word sentences when he could find a thought. He seemed to have a word retrieval problem.

Then he hit kindergarten at an early age of four and a half. I told them about my concern with his speech. They evaluated Jeremy and said he wasn't severe enough to qualify for speech services. After that, I thought everyone else was right.

But I kept insisting to his teacher that something wasn't right. I was going by gut feeling. Gut instinct. I couldn't get this image out of my head: I told Jeremy to take a piece of paper to his room and make his bed. Well, I found him in the bathroom. Obviously, something was wrong. The two aren't even related. But the kindergarten teacher kept denying any problem existed.

Another problem of Jeremy's was the loudness of things, like the lawn mower. It really bothered him. He asked me if I had a volume control on it. He usually stays inside when I'm mowing.

We were starting first grade and still, I had no direction. I didn't know anything. The school didn't tell me anything. Thankfully, I live close to the University of Buffalo. They use a lot of studies with kids in Jeremy's school. I volunteered Jeremy for one of their speech studies, hoping they'd pick up on his problem, whatever it was. That's when they told me they suspected he had an auditory processing problem and referred me to the audiology department.

I'd never heard of APD before. They did a whole battery of tests on him and told me his hearing was fine, but linked me up with a noted audiologist there who works with kids with APD, and she finished the APD testing.

With the conclusion of the tests and clinical history, there was no doubt. He had a "mild case" of APD, but it needed attention. They recommended an FM Trainer, preferred seating, and all that stuff. The FM Trainer is where the teacher wears a microphone, and Jeremy has a headset or speaker on his desk (a receiver) so that he can directly hear what the teacher is saying. He was seen through the summer, Monday through Thursday. Two hours in the morning. It was a godsend. They combined Earobics with individual speech therapy, and auditory training. They taught him strategies to help him, like looking at the person who is speaking. He was at the University of Buffalo for five weeks, and I could see changes right away.

Christina

In a very matter-of-fact way, Christina's mom told me about her struggle to make sure her daughter was accurately diagnosed.

When Christina was born, everything was considered to be normal. She was a very happy and a very, very good baby. By the age of two, however, we started questioning whether or not she could possibly have some type of hearing loss. Her speech didn't seem to be where it should be. And she had chronic ear infections when she was a baby. She'd been hospitalized at six months of age for a severe ear infection.

But the doctor told us that children are different and develop differently and to not worry about it. At age three, Christina was talking, but she still tended to babble and talk more gibberish, not like other kids her age.

We moved to another state at that time, and Christina went to a private preschool. I spoke with the teachers. They and I worked with Christina, and it seemed as if she was doing better. Still, we wondered about a hearing loss.

Another pediatrician told us (after testing in his office) not to be concerned, and again we heard the words, "Different kids develop differently."

She advanced to another year of preschool, and her teacher told me Christina had difficulty sequencing. She was saying "huh?" and "what?" a lot. The biggest thing I noticed was that she couldn't tell me what she did in school that day. Now I know it was short-term memory trouble in addition to her APD.

When Christina got to kindergarten, everything seemed to be going okay. She hadn't received any speech therapy up to that time. We were active Navy and moved a lot. Different pediatricians continually saw Christina, so there wasn't one person who saw her year after year. She still wasn't using whole sentences. She wasn't giving clear messages.

At the end of the first nine weeks, the teacher asked to speak with me. She told me Christina had trouble with oral directions and responding orally to questions. I asked if she thought there was a hearing loss. She wasn't sure, only that Christina might be held back unless she improved. I left the school in tears.

I called my pediatrician and insisted on a hearing test. I also called a free hearing clinic. I took her that afternoon. But the test came back that Christina had 100% hearing acuity in both ears. The pediatrician had also agreed to a referral for "Speech Dysfluency and Auditory Processing." That was the first time I'd seen those words.

But they didn't test for APD, just the hearing test. And again, I was told that everything was fine. So I went to the parent-teacher store and spent a fortune buying games and computer programs that I thought would help her. By the end of kindergarten, she was doing well enough to progress to first grade.

But the teacher in first grade brought the same issues up—trouble following verbal information, following oral directions, responding orally to tests—and now, writing sentences. So I went back to the pediatrician, asking for more audiological testing. Again, they found nothing. After four years of audiological testing, I wasn't very rational. I blew up. I talked to the audiologist and conveyed to her that I thought it had something to do with auditory processing. She asked me to tell her about Christina. Finally, after we talked, she asked me to bring Christina back for an APD evaluation. She said normally kids with this disorder are a little bit quiet, withdrawn, but Christina is very outgoing and self-confident. So she didn't fit the profile socially, although everything else about Christina fit the APD profile very well. I learned you can't depend on the social aspect of the child when APD is considered.

We went back, and Christina was found to have APD. I had very mixed emotions. This was my first baby and there's something wrong with her and she's not normal, but thank God, I finally know what it is. I really felt relief.

Nathan

Nathan's mother is articulate and poised, and happens to be a pediatric occupational therapist. She also became self-reflective as she discussed her son's struggles.

Nathan was a preemie. He was born at 31 weeks gestation and weighed 3 pounds, 11 ounces. He was, thank God, a very healthy preemie, though. When he was an infant, we did notice that he became overstimulated a lot, especially in association with noise. He would shut down in a loud environment. His eyes would kind of blink and roll in another direction. That lasted until he was about six months old. After that, he pretty much developed normally. All of his developmental milestones were within normal limits.

He was very, very verbal, but at almost three, we started noticing some articulation problems. He was leaving off consonants. And another problem they termed "backing," where he would say sounds produced in the front of the mouth like "d" and produce them in back of his mouth like "g," I guess because the sounds sound so much alike. He was in speech therapy for about three months and did spectacularly. Nathan was always easy to remediate.

Nathan was always shy and quiet, a very good little boy. But we noticed that there was something a little different about the way he interacted with people. He got very anxious in social situations. I used to call him "My Third Leg." His first impressions were sometimes misleading to others. Once he knew people, he was fine.

Nathan did very well in preschool. It was a very structured, nurturing religious preschool. He was one of the brightest kids in the class. He started reading at four, visually. We didn't find out until this year that it was purely visual memory. Sight-reading.

But then Nathan entered kindergarten. The public school classroom size was about 33 to 36 children. I knew by Nathan's personality that he would just fall apart in a place like that. So we tried a private school that used a gifted curriculum. Everything was problem solving and critical thinking. And very small classes. He had fifteen kids in his class. It was beautiful. He excelled in kindergarten. He was doing great.

Then in first grade, the one thing we kept noticing was that he couldn't improve on his reading. He was stuck. The sight-reading was failing. And that's when we saw it. He hit a major wall. He went from being one of the highest-level children in preschool and kindergarten to falling way behind. It was a surprise to everyone in the family.

He had such a sweet personality, but within a year, he started getting this nasty tone in his voice. He became very oppositional. I didn't know what was happening. He sounded like a teenager. And I thought, he's really frustrated about something.

So we talked to the teacher. She said, "You know, he's spacing out a bit in class. He's really not giving his best effort." And that wasn't Nathan at all. Nathan was always focused. He worked so hard on things. I knew something wasn't right.

Then we started spelling tests. I'd never seen anything like it. We would study every night. He couldn't get any right. Nothing would stick. Nothing. His language arts papers would come back, targeting opposites and syllables and trying to find main ideas. And nothing. Completely wrong.

We took him for testing at that time. Because I'm a pediatric occupational therapist in the school system, thank God, I had so many contacts to ask who would be good to take Nathan to see. We found a wonderful psychologist who was just head and shoulders above the rest and specialized in pediatric educational testing. He found Nathan's IQ was in the high average range. But there was a three-and-a-half-year delay on—he called it "auditory perception"—but it was really language processing.

I'd heard of APD very vaguely with some of the learning disabled kids that I had worked with. But APD was never looked at as a singular entity. Education threw it in with the other stuff. In fact, this psychologist didn't really diagnose it. His diagnosis for Nathan was "a severe reading disability."

That was when I decided to start hunting because I knew there was still more going on with him. So I started to go online for hours to read as much as I could. There were no books on APD that I could find. I found the LD online web site and started reading the checklist on APD. It was like, "Oh my God, this is my child." It made so much sense. Based on this information I knew that I needed to find professionals who could give me a more complete diagnosis.

By now, Nathan was three-quarters into first grade. I got together a list of recommendations for the school to start working with him in class. Within a week, we saw 100% on spelling tests. We studied two words a night, instead of all ten. We encouraged him to make a picture in his mind. And we asked his teacher to make sure she had his attention when she was speaking to him.

Somehow, we made it through to the end of the year. I took the psychologist's report and asked one of my friends, who is the director of speech pathology at a major university, what I should do. She said, "Depending on what his basic issues are, those issues would determine what would be the best program for him. Are most of his problems in expressive and receptive language or in reading and spelling and verbalizing?"

I said, "Reading, spelling, and verbalizing."

"Then," she said, "Lindamood-Bell."

We went to the Dan Marino Center for Neurological Studies/Miami Children's Hospital Clinics. You know the quarterback for the Miami Dolphins, Dan Marino—it's named after him. They have everything there. It's a wonderful place.

We took him for four hours a day for three weeks, went on vacation for a week, then had him finish with six more weeks. We tried to overlap it with school, but it was too intensive and ended up pulling him out for a few weeks before the end of the year. And that's when we started to see progress. It was kind of like a roller coaster. One week, we'd see huge improvements. The next week, his speech would be almost unintelligible. Things got better. Things got worse. Things got better.

But by the end, it magically came together. Nathan worked very hard. Not once did he wake up and say, "I don't want to go."

The progress he made was remarkable. His reading fluency and rate scores increased by 1.5 years and his comprehension improved by 3 years. He went from requiring numerous modifications in first grade and doing poorly in all language areas to needing almost no modifications in second grade. Audiological testing showed gains from his May testing when he showed a 3.5 year delay in auditory processing, specifically in auditory figure ground, auditory sequencing, auditory memory, and phonemic awareness to showing a mild deficiency in auditory figure ground.

Nathan is back to being a joy. He's excited about learning. I thought after this, I'd have my life back. I thought this would be the end of it all, and we'd be done. Now I don't think it'll be that way. It's consuming. My husband and I went through some grieving. This summer was probably one of the most challenging for us.

We're considering an FM Trainer, based upon the recommendation of an audiologist. We're still trying to decide.

When I'd read Nathan's reports, I'd get nauseated and sob and sob and sob.

But I grew up with a learning disability and at that time, they offered my mother special ed with a class of Down Syndrome children. She refused. So basically, I had to learn on my own how to get through school. And I was honor roll, straight As. I also worked five times as hard as anybody else. I have a lot of faith and know it will be all right.

Missy

Missy and her family live in Singapore, and her mother spoke with me freely and with a wry sense of humor.

Missy is my third daughter. She enjoyed a perfectly normal pregnancy, except for jaundice after birth. But it resolved after she was put under the bilirubin light. And she was a big baby: 9.1 pounds. I think there is a familial pattern to all this. My youngest brother had real problems. He used to say it physically hurt him to write. Again, he was very, very smart. But he didn't do well in school.

I guess the thing that was unusual about Missy was the way she learned how to speak. She would have these sentences made up of syllables, but they didn't mean anything, and in the middle of it there might be a word. So you'd get jibber-jabber, then a word, then more jibber-jabber. I remember one time when Missy was three; she was angry with her sisters and came to tell me. Her cadence was right, her tone was right. It was unintelligible. She made communication just fine; there just wasn't any-body who could understand it. She made up her own language. Recep-tively, you didn't want to have to get into any sophisticated concepts because you knew it wasn't going to go anywhere. The more concrete the better. Missy was the only one of my kids to watch a television show or a film repeatedly.

By now, we lived in the UK. They're not real up on APD. In some ways, they were ahead of the United States in that they had identified what they call dyslexia, which is this big umbrella term that takes in all kinds of reading difficulties. They didn't separate out APD at all, at least at that particular time.

They usually started kids reading at age three. The teacher knew some-thing was off and suggested a psychologist to figure out if there was a learn-ing problem. I mean, Missy would work on phonetic reading and she would sound out "d" "o" "g," and look at you and say, "cat." She just didn't get it.

We had her hearing tested when she was five, and the results were fine. The psychologist said her IQ was average, and that she might have an auditory processing problem, but he didn't diagnose anything until age seven. The teacher helped us and hooked us up with a trained dyslexic tutor. Missy made some gains, and when she was seven, we moved to Sin-gapore and into an American school.

The American school held a meeting and told us she was fine and I thought, "yeah, right." The teacher agreed with us and said the meeting was too soon and that "something wasn't clicking with her." Her speech was normal by then, except that (even now) she didn't get pronouns right. She couldn't pick up new words quickly either. Missy's teacher was the one who got on the Internet and found APD. She asked us if we'd ever heard of it. She gave me a checklist, and I said, "This is it. It matches Missy to-tally." I mean, it wasn't a diagnosis, but it gave me a direction to go in.

The following summer, we took her to the States for complete testing. Her IQ was found to be 130. We hooked into Fast ForWord and Step 4word the following summer when we returned to the States. Missy also continued with the tutor. She was now close to fourth grade.

But in the middle of all this, we had a complete audiological workup just before returning to Singapore. The audiologist noted: "Interhemi-

spheric integration (linguistic labeling of temporal patterns, durational cues, auditory and nonauditory information); and left-hemispheric auditory closure skills."

Now *it got into an* Outer Limits *kind of thing because, after all the tutoring and computer programs, we took her back after fourth grade and one year later, after repeat audiological testing and a brain scan and a complete workup, he came back and said, "She's perfectly normal."*

We'd also started her on an FM Trainer six months prior to this testing. It was a real breakthrough for Missy. It had a headset for Missy to use, and all of a sudden, if you looked at what happened with her grades and with her writing and everything, it all leaped forward. It was unbelievable. Like "Welcome to Holland"—you know that metaphor about having a disabled child—only in reverse. My thing is that I want her to perform to her potential. Not to be normal, but to be the best she can be.

Summary

Parents know when the child needs them, as well as the help of others to prepare for life. Children with APD may very well have lifelong issues to deal with, but information is power. Coping skills develop when the individual knows what strengths and weaknesses he or she possesses. I believe there is much to learn about APD, much to understand. I also believe there is much to celebrate on behalf of our children.

One Year Later

I'D HEARD THAT FIRST AND SECOND GRADES MARK THE END of the early elementary years. Third grade, it was whispered, had multiplication tables, more heavy-duty reading. Textbooks. Real tests. And report cards with letter grades. Although Ben was now equipped with his own set of oars, I wondered if he would know how to pull himself forward.

I didn't want to waste those precious summer months between second and third grade, so I signed Ben up for a science day camp, a two-night outdoorsy camp, and weekly piano lessons for both boys. Three days a week we tackled summer "bridge workbook" exercises. Ben went back to Earobics Step 1 since he'd never completed it. I wanted to assess how he would do on the games, particularly the one with increasing background noise. He breezed through it, finishing the program in about three weeks. The boys and I visited the library regularly, and John read with Ben every night.

All that I'd heard about third grade was true, and as I looked at the stack of books piled on Ben's new desk at the parents' open house in the fall, I felt sick to my stomach. The teacher, Miss Gilbert, nodded to John and me. I slipped her my APD handout that included a description of the disorder and classroom recommendations, with extra copies for the teacher's assistant and his new speech therapist. I felt I was starting over and missed Mrs. Perkins terribly.

The first few months were bumpy for Ben. When we sat down for his IEP conference in the fall, Miss Gilbert told me that he was continually asking for help and seemed worried about pleasing her and the other teachers. Some of the difficulties stemmed from understanding the directions of what was wanted on the assignment; some of it was difficulty with the content. But I wondered if some of it was Ben's lack of confidence. Although Ben now had his own set of oars, he was afraid to use them.

During the conference, his teacher, speech therapist, and I decided Ben needed to try at least once on his own before asking for help. His new speech therapist decided to integrate some of his social studies and science curriculum into their speech therapy sessions, held twice weekly. And he was still in Reading Lab for support in language arts.

That night, John and I tried to explain it to Ben. He shook his head, his glasses stained from recesses playing basketball with the other boys. "I don't understand sometimes. I need help."

"That's okay. They'll help you, Ben. But first you have to try on your own."

"They won't help me anymore?"

"Yes, they'll help you. But first you have to try."

"Is my teacher mad at me?"

"No. Not at all."

"What if I don't do so good? What if I get a D or F?" He clearly understood the stakes.

"Then we'll figure out why you got the D or the F and go from there."

"You still help me?"

"I help you every night, don't I?" I paused. "You're really smart, Ben."

"I am?"

"Oh, yes. Very smart."

He looked at both of us. "Okay, I try first, but if I don't understand, the teacher help me?"

"Yes, she will, Ben."

IT TOOK SEVERAL MONTHS OF REASSURING BEN IT WAS OKAY TO fail—at times. And struggling at first didn't mean he wouldn't eventually get it. He had to learn to have patience, to trust himself. And me. He came home with some Ds and Fs and watched me closely for my reaction. I'd ask if he tried his best, to which he always nodded vigorously. I'd shrug my shoulders and assure him we'd go over the paper that night so he would understand next time.

On his IEP plan, I'd requested an extra set of textbooks for home use, and we opened them on many nights. Miss Gilbert communicated areas that were tricky for Ben, just as Mrs. Perkins had done. There were study cards and sheets distributed to the entire class to help the students prepare for the social studies and science tests. Using these study guides and the textbooks, I made practice tests for these subjects. Ben and I went over how to decode multiple-choice questions, and how to carefully read "True" and "False" statements. During the exams, the teachers supported his efforts, particularly on the short essay. Slowly and gradually, they stepped back.

Ben began to trust that it was okay to try. He learned that I was still going to help steer, and Miss Gilbert kept him on course at school. He started to take the chance of not succeeding, and by doing so, began to succeed. Near the end of the final quarter, I wanted to touch base with Miss Gilbert, whom I'd learned to appreciate. She had a dry humor and relaxed demeanor with the kids. Ben called her "silly," and I could tell he liked her a lot. I'd popped in to ask her a question about a project at the school and said, "Ben says he's doing more work by himself."

"He sure is. So what he gets on his report card, he's earned himself."

I looked at her sharply, but then saw a hint of a grin on her face. "He seems to be doing okay."

She nodded and turned briefly to check on the class from the doorway where we stood. "He's doing very well."

I COULD TELL BEN'S SMALL SUCCESSES HAD ROCKETED HIS SELF-confidence. He continued to routinely get 100% on his spelling tests and in the high 90s for math computation tests. Reading Lab had also focused on his math word problems to try to help him understand what computation the problem called for. Ben would now get in the car and tell me what he was able to do independently and what he needed help with.

Ben was also taking the initiative more at home. I'd purchased a fifteen-dollar children's program on keyboarding/typing. He'd stuck with it and got the basics down. He started to write stories about a character called Little Bill and his camp adventures. He continued with Cub Scouts and worked hard on patches and other decorations for his shirt.

I was also adapting to Annie and Annie to me. The baby from the two-dimensional pictures in Calcutta was sitting on my lap, refusing to drink her bottle and kicking me. The love of the idea of having a baby transformed into loving this baby. My heart felt like an hourglass, filling with grains of sand as my feelings for this feisty, sweet infant took hold. And her love for me grew as well; she began preferring my presence to everyone else's, crying when I left the room. She started to walk and babble, and would run up to me to hug my leg. To earn a child's love is like arriving in heaven.

I watched Annie's milestones closely, too, and found myself saying things during her well-child checks like, "Her receptive abilities are on target developmentally. She can follow one-step directions, and her preverbal utterances have also increased appropriately." I'd become a Collective Mom who knew the lingo.

Peter finished kindergarten and Mrs. Minett gushed about what a good year it had been for him. How he'd matured, she thought, because of Annie's presence in the family. He was reading phonics books and doing basic math problems. He was ready to join Ben at the public school next year as a first grader.

Just after spring break, I picked Ben up from school, and from out of his backpack he took a blue sheet of paper marked: "To the Parents of Ben Thompson." It was Ben's final midterm report card. I pulled the car over onto one of the many gravel drives in the area.

I opened the blue piece of paper.

All As with the exception of one B+. Miss Gilbert wrote: "Ben is strong academically. He continues to work more and more independently. He is completely on grade level in all areas. He is social and a very well behaved little boy who has friends."

On grade level in all areas.

I kept reading the words over and over, not because I didn't believe them, but because—for now and for the first time in his life—Ben was caught up.

"Ben, you almost got straight As." I couldn't remember the last time I had smiled so hard that my facial muscles hurt.

"I know. Miss Gilbert said we could look." He smiled just as happily back at me.

"I'm so proud of you, Ben. So very proud."

As soon as I got home, I paged John—so different from the many pages I'd done just as urgently.

After I told him the news, he said, "That's fantastic." We left unspoken that this precious moment was a celebration for us as parents. Our boy had done good.

"Are you almost finished there?" I asked. John had stayed at the hospital, this job, and had found his niche.

"Almost. I'll see you soon."

"We ought to do something special, for the whole family."

"I agree. Let's think about it."

I reviewed the rest of Ben's work that Miss Gilbert sent home in a "graded papers" folder every day. There was a picture that Ben had drawn and colored. All the family was present, and Ben sat at a computer. There were two stacks of books and an arrow pointing to them. He'd written: "Books. When I grow up, I'm going to be a writer."

After putting Annie up for her afternoon nap, I called, "Ben, time to do homework." I leaned over to kiss him on the cheek. "I told you you were smart."

He smiled as he sharpened his pencil and opened his English book on the kitchen table. I started to sit down.

"No, Mom. I want to try to do it by myself. Is that okay?"

"That's fine, Benny. That's just fine."

"But you stay here."

"I'll be right here." And as I walked over to start dinner— wondering what was in the freezer that I'd neglected to thaw—I thought about that water, once such a deep dark purple. I thought about the small boat that barely kept me from drowning, and I watched my little boy start to row.

Resources

Organizations

NCAPD (National Coalition for Auditory Processing
   Disorders, Inc.)
Founded by Debbie Wood and Dr. Jay Lucker
P.O. Box 11810
Jacksonville, Florida 32239-1810
www.ncapd.org
Includes a state-by-state APD referral network

ASHA (American Speech-Language-Hearing Association)
10801 Rockville Pike
Rockville, Maryland 20852
(888) 321-ASHA
www.asha.org

American Academy of Audiology
8300 Greensboro Drive
Suite 750
McLean, Virginia 22102
(800) AAA-2336
(703) 790-8466
www.audiology.org

CASLPA (Canadian Association of Speech-Language
   Pathologists and Audiologists)
2006-130 Albert Street
Ottawa, Ontario K1P 5G4
(613) 567-9968
E-mail: caslpa@caslpa.ca

Recommended Reading

Bellis, Teri James. *Assessment and Management of Central Auditory Processing Disorders in the Educational Setting from Science to Practice.* San Diego: Singular Publishing Group, 1996.

Bellis, Teri James. *When the Brain Can't Hear: Unraveling the Mystery of Auditory Processing Disorder.* New York: Pocket Books, 2002.

Chermak, Gail D., Frank E. Musiek, and Chie Higuchi Craig. *Central Auditory Processing Disorders: New Perspectives.* San Diego: Singular Press, 1997.

Ferre, Jeanne M. *Processing Power: A Guide to CAPD Assessment and Management.* San Antonio: Communication Skill Builders/The Psychological Corporation, 1997.

Hamaguchi, Patricia McAleer. *Childhood Speech, Language and Listening Problems: What Every Parent Should Know.* New York: John Wiley & Sons, Inc. 1995.

Kelly, Dorothy A. *Central Auditory Processing Disorder: Strategies for Use with Children and Adolescents.* San Antonio: The Psychological Corporation, 1999.

Masters, M. Gay, Nancy A. Stecker, and Jack Katz. *Central Auditory Processing Disorders: Mostly Management.* Boston: Allyn and Bacon, 1998.

Corporations/Products

Scientific Learning Corporation (Fast ForWord Reading and
Language Products)
300 Frank H. Ogawa Plaza
Suite 500
Oakland, California 94612-2040
(888) 665-9707
*Cross Train is now available to parents as an option to obtaining a
service provider.*
www.scientificlearning.com

Lindamood-Bell Learning Processes (Learning Programs,
including the LiPS and V/V)
416 Higuera Street
San Luis Obispo, California 93401
(800) 233-1819
*Learning centers are located throughout the United States (including
Indianapolis, Indiana) and abroad.*
www.lblp.com

Cognitive Concepts (Earobics Step 1 and 2)
990 Grove Street
Evanston, Illinois 60201
(888) 328-8199
(847) 328-8099 (Outside U.S.)
www.earobics.com and www.cogcon.com